Andrew Wilson is a Registered O̶____ four years' training in London at the British College of Naturopathy and Osteopathy. For the last 13 years he has had his own busy practice in Tauranga, New Zealand. He is a past President of the New Zealand Register of Osteopaths and was the N.Z.R.O. Registered Osteopath of the Year in 1991.

He has a particular interest in posture and sports injuries. Among his other interests he includes: running, kayaking and wine tasting.

The front cover illustrates problems:
Neither sitter comfortably has feet on
floor; in order to achieve certain stability, they are in chairs with "specially"
designed sloping seats which tips them
+ their circu- lation forward
+ down.
Why can't table be lower?
And I disagree
with castors-
In reality the man could probably
easily have his feet planted on floor.

ARE YOU SITTING COMFORTABLY?

A self-help guide for sufferers of
back pain, neck strain, headaches,
RSI, and other associated health
problems

Andrew Wilson

OPTIMA

An Optima Book

First published in the United Kingdom by Optima in 1994

Copyright © 1994 Andrew Wilson

The moral right of the author has been asserted

A CIP catalogue for this book
is available from the British Library

ISBN 0 356 21060 X

Typeset by Solidus (Bristol) Limited
Printed and bound in Great Britain by
Clays Ltd, St. Ives PLC

Optima
A division of
Little, Brown and Company (UK)
Brettenham House
Lancaster Place
London WC2E 7EN

Contents

Acknowledgements

There are many people who have made important contributions to the development of this book. James Fisk seemed to be asking the right questions. A.C. Mandal had some of the right answers long before me. Dennis Zacharkow, Etienne Grandjean, Tom Bendix and Steven Pheasant have done excellent research in this area, and their work has provided important milestones in the development of my thoughts. There are many others whose research and writings have contributed to this tree of knowledge. My thanks to them.

Jenny Wallace has done a superb job with the illustrations. Richard Carruthers and Sheryl Walker have provided valuable support and proof-reading skills. The headmaster and pupils of Mount Maunganui College have helped with research and illustrations. My family, friends and colleagues have supported and encouraged my endeavours, especially my wife, Elspeth, whose understanding and typing skills have graced this project. My grateful thanks to my patients, they are perhaps the best teachers of all.

This book is dedicated to those people who have the courage to ask the difficult questions.

Preface

> Whatever you do, or think you can do, begin it.
> Boldness has genius, power and magic in it.
> Begin it now.
>
> Goethe

I came to realise that what I regarded as one of the major causes of musculoskeletal distress seemed to be largely ignored by many people. I was convinced that improved awareness of the sitting posture could benefit a great many people and help reduce the rapidly escalating incidence of joint problems.

There has been good-quality research outlining improvements in sitting posture using such things as forward sloping seats and backward tilting desks, but these seem to have been largely ignored by many health agencies and influential authorities. This information needed to be presented in a form that would be approachable for the health consumer, who in my experience is often well-motivated and keen to learn methods of improving health and fitness. It needed to be written by someone who was used to dealing with joint problems, and the pain and discomfort associated with them; with an emphasis on self-help and personal responsibility.

I began to realise that the rapid move toward computer-isation of the workplace was leaving many people in pain and discomfort as they came to grips with the working methods of the new technology. The problems arising from the repetitive strain of computer work seem to be poorly understood and few resources are available for the prevention and treatment of these problems. Even as I write this debate rages following Judge Prosser's decision in the High Court that RSI is meaningless and has no place in the medical books.

There is a shortage of good-quality information. Knowledge and understanding of health issues provide the background to make the important decisions required to improve health status. Good-quality health information is important to develop understanding of the issues, and to make the appropriate choices. In the early chapters of this book I have tried to present the background information that leads to a good understanding of the issues, while the latter portion explores the solutions. If you are feeling impatient to implement some of the self-help techniques, you might like to start at chapter 5 and return to the earlier chapters to gain the understanding subsequently.

This book has been written to provide the type of information I would like my patients to have. I hope you find it helpful.

Andrew Wilson, November 1993

Introduction

Are you sitting comfortably?

Are you sure?

How long will you be comfortable?

Do you know the difference between good and bad posture?

These are questions we rarely ask ourselves. When we consider that about half the population spend over 70 per cent of their waking day sitting, and when we consider that the consequences of prolonged sitting include pain, disability, health problems, time off work, lost production and increased health care costs, perhaps we should be thinking about the answers.

People have always sat down. It gives rest to the ankles, knees and hips, and the muscles involved in stabilising these joints. Sitting uses less energy than standing. Sitting significantly changes posture and places considerable stresses on the spine, a part of the body that is not designed to cope with continual postural stress.

Good posture and good-quality seating were less important in the past when sitting periods were brief and tissues under stress had plenty of time to recover. The alteration in our lifestyle, particularly over the last 100 years – the demands of the education system; the advent of machinery and labour-saving devices that have replaced most manual work; the increasing adoption of sedentary leisure activities such as television, video and computer games – have completely altered our way of life. We spend long periods sitting, with very little alteration in our posture.

Let's consider an example. On an average day an adolescent sleeps an estimated nine hours and is awake for 15 hours. On a school day the 15 wakeful hours might be broken down as follows:

	Active hours	*Sitting hours*
Dressing and preparing for school	½	
Travel		1
School		5½
School breaks	½	
Meals		1
Homework		1
Leisure (television, computer, video, reading)		3
Active leisure	1	
Miscellaneous	½	½
Prepare for bed	½	
Total in hours	3	12
Total as a percentage of time	20%	80%

This young person has spent 80 per cent of his or her day sitting despite spending one hour's active leisure after school. If we did a similar analysis for a sedentary worker it would show a similar or higher percentage of time spent sitting. Even the active sportsperson would be unlikely to spend more than an extra five hours per week physically active (running or squash five times, or one game of football and two long practices) and would still be spending 75 per cent of wakeful time sitting overall.

Anthropologists have long been of the opinion that the spinal problems that plague mankind are because we are designed to be walking on all fours. Let's examine this theory. It is estimated that 80 per cent of the population suffer from back pain at some point in their lives. This ratio has dramatically increased during the last 100 years and is continuing to increase. One would expect with evolution that we would be gradually adapting to the bipedal posture as we have been on two feet for several million years. This is clearly not the case as the incidence of back pain and musculoskeletal problems continues to rise dramatically. What is it that we have been doing that has caused this marked increase? I believe it is the continuing and increasing use of the sitting posture. In historical terms this has been a lifestyle revolution.

DOES SITTING AFFECT CHILDREN?

My interest in seating and the sitting posture was first aroused when I was researching Scheuermann's Disease (SD), a degenerative condition that affects the spine of teenagers. I came across a study that showed the incidence was dramatically increasing. In an assessment of 500 17 and 18 year olds, it was found that 56.3 per cent of the boys and 30.3 per cent of the girls had x-ray evidence of SD: an astonishing incidence in otherwise healthy children. The researchers concluded: 'In the absence of possible dynamic stress factors it is suggested that prolonged sitting may be an important factor in the pathogenesis of end plate breakdown and thus Scheuermann's disease.' This topic is covered in greater detail in chapter 3.

Could it be that a high proportion of children are condemned to a life of back pain because we force them to adopt a poor sitting position every day? The evidence certainly suggests that this is the case.

As an osteopath I devised a treatment protocol to treat the symptoms of SD when they arose. This treatment met with some success and in most cases alleviated the symptoms. However, the underlying degenerative changes could not be reversed, and the permanently damaged spine remained weakened and likely to present recurrent problems.

The most effective approach to the problem of SD in young people would be prevention: to avoid the build up of spinal stresses that create the degenerative changes. This led me to study the human posture; how it changes in the sitting position; the ergonomics of chair design; the ergonomics of the desk or 'work station'; and other lifestyle management factors. The conclusion I came to was that the sitting posture is a major cause of pain, discomfort and disease in our society. We cannot stop people sitting, our twentieth-century lifestyle demands it. We can, however, ensure that with good advice, good seating, good posture and good management, we can dramatically reduce the incidence and minimise the effects of this lifestyle revolution.

ERGONOMICS
The science of adapting working conditions to the human being.

All sectors of society, from young children to the elderly, from office workers to truck drivers, could benefit from increased awareness of their sitting posture and ways to improve and effectively manage it.

When we consider the scale of this lifestyle revolution, it is surprising how little is understood of its consequences and how few resources are harnessed to study and minimise its effects. Most postural advice is of the 'sit up straight' variety. This book will show that sitting up straight on a horizontal seat is quite a difficult posture to maintain because the muscles soon become fatigued. It is also very difficult to read and write effectively at a conventional desk while sitting up straight because the visual angle and distance are very poor.

CAN SITTING CAUSE BACK PAIN?

When a person suffers a serious back injury, one of the most difficult things is to sit for any length of time. They are usually more comfortable standing or lying. The pain on sitting is usually the last symptom to resolve, due to the extra pressure it causes in the spine. This can be a serious problem for people whose work requires a lot of sitting and can result in prolonged periods of time off work.

I often found that when these patients borrowed forward-tilting or 'kneeler chairs' they were able to sit for longer periods than on a conventional chair. As a result they were able to return to work sooner, with reduced pain levels and without risk of a relapse. For many of them this was a temporary measure, until they were sufficiently recovered to resume their normal seating, though a significant number chose to continue using the forward-tilting or kneeler chairs because they found them more comfortable. This demonstrated to me that the type of chair that people sit on can have a significant effect on posture, and can determine whether a person will develop back or other joint injuries.

I began to realise that many serious spinal injuries were produced by very minor events, such as bending down to tie a shoe lace or sweeping the floor. There had to be another reason why otherwise healthy people could develop a serious spinal injury from such an insignificant event.

The discs in the spine, the shock-absorbing pads between the vertebrae, have very few nerve endings compared to other tissues. This means they can often be under considerable strain without giving any warning signs, such as pain or stiffness. Continuous strain under these conditions squashes and narrows the disc, rendering it less effective: until the final straw – a minor event that can produce a serious injury. For many people it is the long periods of sitting that weakens their spine and allows serious injuries to occur.

Thus, the type of seats, the way we sit and the way we manage the sitting that we do can be important factors in the production and management of spinal injuries.

REPETITIVE STRAIN INJURIES

In recent years there has been a dramatic increase in neck, shoulder and arm problems in sedentary workers. Research has shown that some occupational groups have a 50 to 60 per cent incidence of these problems. There is a markedly higher incidence in keyboard workers compared to traditional clerical workers. It has been established that the increased incidence is related to doing repetitive work in a fixed sitting posture. Hence the name – repetitive strain injury (RSI).

There are a number of interrelated variables that will determine whether a person will get RSI. The main influences are: the working posture of the upper half of the body; the work station design; and working habits. Later in the book I will explain these factors and show that with good posture, good work station design and sensible work management with regular breaks, these problems can be prevented and their effects minimised.

PRINCIPLES OF GOOD POSTURE

Just as people are all different shapes and sizes, there is no one perfect sitting posture that suits everybody. It depends on the individual body type, individual preferences, age, medical history and the task performed. The seat is merely an interface between the individual and the task at hand.

There may not be the perfect chair, but there are good postural principles. These will be clearly outlined, so the reader may choose the sitting posture that best suits them in their own environment. Once a good sitting posture has been found, there are other relevant factors to be considered, including: regular alterations to posture; regular breaks; preventing repetitive strain injuries. This book will explain the importance of these aspects and enable the reader to make the time spent sitting as productive as possible, while avoiding the detrimental effects of the prolonged sitting posture.

SELF-HELP

The book will detail the common problems that occur as a result of the sitting posture, with advice on how to treat, manage and prevent these problems.

1

The history of sitting

We enjoy sitting. It gives some parts of our body a rest. Our ankles, knees and hips, and the muscles which stabilise these joints are no longer weight bearing and are able to relax. Our postural muscles which continually fine tune our balance and work to keep us upright are given a period of relief. Overall the body uses considerably less energy to sit, than to stand or walk. However, there is usually some extra work to be done by the spinal muscles to stabilise the altered posture when we are sitting.

All societies have adopted the sitting posture, though it has been freely adapted according to the culture, the social status, the type of clothes, the purpose, and the materials and skills available to manufacture the actual seat.

CULTURAL VARIATIONS

Many people in Eastern and Middle Eastern societies sit with their legs arranged horizontally, as in the lotus or Buddha position. This is a comfortable and stable sitting position, usually used for relaxing or contemplating rather than a working posture.

Another common position in some societies is squatting. Here the knees and hips are locked in full flexion and require little muscle power to hold them in this position. There are two variations on this. The first has the back supported against a tree or fence, with the buttocks resting on the ground. The second shows free squatting with no support, with the weight transferred from the buttocks to the heels and the arms frequently resting on the knees which provide a secondary support.

Both methods of squatting involve a reverse of the normal lumbar curve which is considered poor posture. They both have mechanisms where much of the weight is transferred from the spine to other supporting structures which reduces the load transmitted through the spinal column.

It is worth noting that many of these societies have a stature that is smaller and leaner than their Western counterparts, and so the forces transmitted through their joints would be a good deal less. It is interesting to consider whether the problems associated with sitting may be in part due to the gradual increase in the size and weight of recent generations, combined with the reduction in muscle tone as a consequence of our sedentary lifestyles. These combine to place considerably increased forces through joints that have not been able to adapt to these changed lifestyles.

The squatting and lotus postures require training from an early age to develop the joint laxity required to hold them in a relaxed manner for long periods of time. It is unrealistic to expect most adult Westerners to assume them habitually. My own attempts at the lotus have proven futile and uncomfortable. Supported squatting was a bit easier though my feet developed pins and needles within 10 minutes. It could be a useful posture when working at ground level, such as weeding the garden.

SITTING AS A STATUS SYMBOL

Sitting on a raised platform, such as a bench, stool or chair, confers an element of superiority over the other members of a society who would usually be seated lower and are symbolically inferior. This superior position would be enhanced by an upright, erect posture which symbolised dignity and purpose. As the sitting posture developed in societies, it was designed to enhance the social status of the sitter whose function it was to rule. The upright sitting posture developed as a means of exercising authority and effective communication rather than as a working posture. The design of seating emphasised this role. There are a number of descriptions which illustrate the authority invested in the seated person: chairman, seat of learning, parliamentary seat and throne.

The Greeks recognised the distinction between sitting for authority and sitting for relaxation, and developed designs incorporating a curved back support and contoured seat which aided comfort and repose. The Greeks and Romans ate their meals reclining on low couches avoiding sitting altogether. Subsequent European cultures have sacrificed comfort preferring to sit upright with the flat seat and vertical chair back. Most household seating consisted of benches or stools which were pulled out at meal times. In the late seventeenth century the easy chair began to appear and offered an opportunity to relax after completing the day's tasks.

DEVELOPMENT OF THE MODERN SITTING POSTURE

In the Victorian era, the industrialisation of society and the creation of an education system produced a whole new demand for seating. Office work became commonplace and

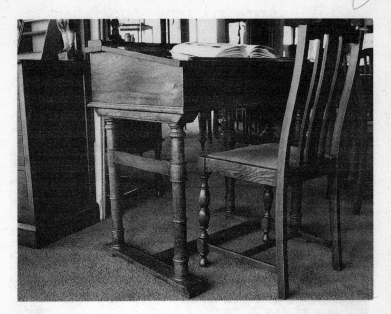

Fig. 1.1 Desks from the late Victorian period. These are examples of excellent furniture design for tasks involving reading and writing.

sitting throughout the working day became a new phenomenon. This was not sitting for authority or relaxation but as a working posture. The Victorian sitting position was a formal one, sitting bolt upright and displaying discipline and dignity in so doing. This was particularly the case for women who were constrained by corsets and crinolines. The furniture design of this period reflected these formal postures. The chairs and tables were higher than is now normal, and sloping desks allowed people to write with a straight back and head held erect. There are some excellent examples of furniture design from this period, when furniture was designed with good posture as a priority.

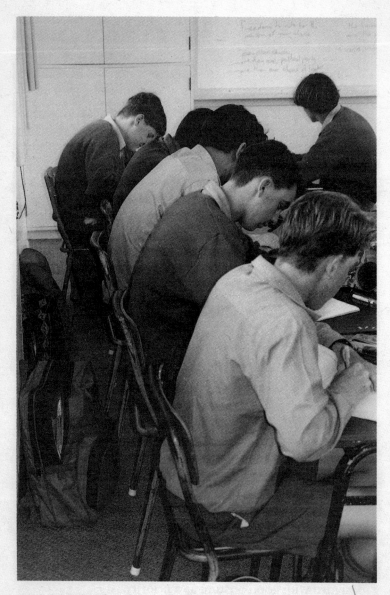

Fig. 1.2 Modern furniture in schools encourages dreadful posture.

The twentieth century has seen a gradual relaxation of society's formalities and this has been reflected in our furniture design and our more relaxed approach to the sitting posture. There is no single posture that is regarded as socially acceptable and chair design allows a wide range of positions. Many of these can be unhealthy and damaging if prolonged.

Furniture design has become influenced by aesthetic and technical demands rather than by postural considerations. We have had to learn to adapt to the seating provided rather than the seating being designed for us. In schools and other institutions where unit cost is the main criterion, the low chair and low horizontal desk have become the norm. This not only allows but encourages dreadful posture. It is a great shame that we allow our young people to develop such poor physiques by providing them with low quality seating.

In the last 20 years there has been renewed interest in sitting positions. The computerisation of the workplace and the health problems associated with prolonged sitting in a fixed posture have encouraged a new area of research into the design and manufacture of good-quality seating and work environments. This is starting to be appreciated by private sector businesses which are quick to realise that content, pain-free employees will be well motivated, more productive and absent less often.

In future years I hope we will see increasing co-operation between furniture designers, ergonomists and therapists – with continual reference to the user of the finished product. Let us design furniture for the people that use it.

2

Can sitting affect your health?

Our bodies are dynamic structures. They adapt and change according to their environment. The way we use them can influence their structure and their ability to function effectively. Our modern sedentary lifestyle, and the increasing amount of sitting that it requires, can have profound effects on our different body systems. These can have long-term health implications. In this chapter we will identify some of the problems that can arise from prolonged sitting.

CIRCULATION

One of the difficulties of sitting is its complete lack of physical activity. Exercise has a very beneficial effect on our circulatory system. The heart is a muscle. It responds to exercise by becoming stronger and functioning more efficiently. A lack of exercise produces a weakening of the heart and a rise in the heartbeat (pulse) as it compensates for its lack of strength by contracting more often to circulate the blood. A relatively weak heart, from lack of exercise, has difficulty coping with an increased level of activity when the need arises, such as walking uphill or climbing stairs.

Regular aerobic exercise increases the amount of high-density lipoproteins in the blood. These reduce the viscosity of the blood (i.e. stickiness) and are an active protective factor against heart disease. A lack of exercise has the reverse effect, increasing the number of low-density lipoproteins (LDL), increasing the viscosity of the blood and increasing the workload on the heart. The increased viscosity of the blood and the presence of LDLs are factors that lead to deposits on the artery walls. These deposits are known as atheroma and are part of a disease process known as atherosclerosis. The blockage of the artery walls affects the circulation and is the major cause of heart attacks and strokes. Thus the lack of exercise our sedentary lifestyle encourages is a major risk factor in arterial disease and its consequences. It provides another powerful reason for people who lead inactive lifestyles to make a point of doing regular aerobic exercise.

Venous return

Muscular contraction has a powerful pumping effect on the circulation. It forces blood out of the muscles back through the veins towards the heart. One of the important muscle pumps is the soleus, often described as the second heart. The soleus is situated deep in the calf and has a major function in walking, running and all foot and ankle movements. It is a postural muscle that is highly active in all standing and walking postures, and largely inactive in sitting postures. The veins within the muscle contain

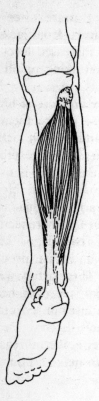

Fig. 2.1 The soleus muscle acts as a powerful vascular pump, assisting the return of blood to the heart.

Fig. 2.2 Pressure from the seat can affect the return of circulation in the femoral veins.

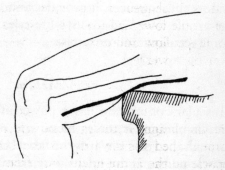

cavities with strong valves just below them. The blood pools in the cavities and the contraction of the soleus forces the blood back toward the heart.

The absence of the soleus pump in the sitting position allows the blood to pool in the veins, increasing the pressure on the vein walls. This can be both a cause and an irritating factor of varicose veins and can significantly increase the risk of venous thrombosis – blood clotting in the veins of the leg. There is a risk of these clots travelling to the lung and causing a pulmonary embolism – a potentially fatal blockage.

The return of venous blood from the lower limbs can also be hindered by the pressure on the femoral veins in the back of the thighs, from sitting near the edge of the seat. This can put pressure on the vein wall, increasing the resistance to the venous return of blood. There are research papers that correlate the length and type of sitting posture with increased foot swelling, reduction in temperature in the feet and discomfort in the feet and lower legs.

Regular changes in posture while sitting, with contraction of the lower limb muscles, have a beneficial effect on the blood flow and improves the venous return of blood from the lower legs.

BREATHING

The diaphragm is the main muscle of breathing. It is a dome-shaped muscle lying at the bottom of the lungs, separating the abdominal cavity from the chest cavity. A contraction of this muscle increases the volume of the chest cavity, sucking air into the lungs. A relaxation of the muscle returns the ribs and lungs back to their original diameters, expelling the air.

As the diaphragm contracts, sucking air into the chest, it

increases the abdominal pressure by pressing against the abdominal cavity and, in combination with the stomach muscles, reducing the abdominal space. This acts as a powerful muscle pump. The abdominal organs are richly endowed with blood supply, and the piston-like action of the diaphragm squeezes blood from the abdominal cavity and sucks it back to the heart in the chest cavity.

The primary function of the diaphragm is breathing, and in the absence of physical exertion it operates without any assistance from the chest muscles. It has an important secondary function as a vascular pump, helping to return blood from the abdominal cavity and organs to the heart.

The change in posture, from an upright posture when standing to the more usual slouched posture when sitting, makes it very difficult for the diaphragm to work effectively. The normal sitting posture crowds the thorax and compresses the rib cage, reducing the diameter of the lungs. It squashes the abdominal cavity, reducing the ability of the diaphragm to descend, and together with the complete relaxation of the stomach muscles, its effectiveness in both its respiratory and muscle pump roles is reduced.

The brain requires a large amount of oxygen to function effectively, and approximately 25 per cent of the heart's output of oxygen-rich blood is destined for it. The handicap to breathing and circulation caused by the slouched sitting posture makes it difficult for the body to meet with these demands. Concentration can be very difficult to maintain when sitting for long periods simply because the brain is not being bathed sufficiently in freshly oxygenated blood to work effectively.

The more upright the sitting posture, the better the quality of breathing, circulation and oxygenation of the brain. This produces better concentration and improved efficiency. Regular movement – not just while sitting, but getting up and moving about – gets the muscle pumps working and the blood flow surging with freshly oxygenated blood. It wakes you up! It's amazing how a seemingly difficult problem seems to have an easy solution after a bit of exercise.

Proper diaphragmatic breathing is an essential part of good health. The sitting posture tends to encourage bad breathing habits, using some of the less efficient chest muscles. Proper diaphragmatic breathing is described in chapter 10.

DIGESTION

The sitting posture crowds the abdominal cavity. As outlined above, this affects the circulation to the organs, hindering the general digestive process. The crowding of the intestines affects the passage of foodstuff through the digestive tract, leading to a general sluggishness. This can cause or aggravate constipation, diverticulitis (inflamed pockets through the muscular wall of the colon) and malabsorption syndromes. A number of studies have shown an increased risk of bowel cancer in sedentary workers. It is particularly important to avoid a poor sitting posture following a meal. The crowded abdominal cavity shows a general increase in pressure as the abdominal organs try to fit into a smaller space. This can create a problem with gastric reflux, where the highly acidic contents of the stomach are pushed up into the oesophagus (the food pipe from the mouth to the stomach). The oesophagus is not designed to cope with this level of acidity and this causes the discomfort known as heartburn. Heartburn can occur on its own or can be a complication of hiatus hernia. A hiatus hernia is where a portion of the stomach is pushed up through the diaphragm into the chest cavity.

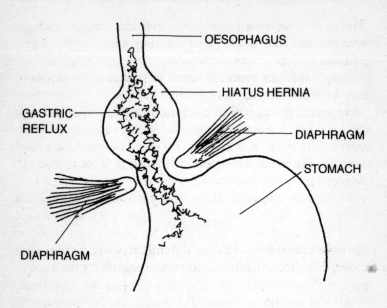

Fig. 2.3 Increased abdominal pressure can lead to hiatus hernia and gastric reflux.

OSTEOPOROSIS

Osteoporosis is a reduction in bone density. It affects mainly post-menopausal women. It is a serious health problem because of the increased risk of bone fractures. These occur mainly at the hip, wrist and spinal vertebrae. Currently about 12 per cent of women develop hip fractures, of which about 10 to 20 per cent die following the fall. This is increasing in incidence, and it is estimated that at current rates of increase, by the year 2016, 24 per cent of women will suffer a fractured hip before the age of 85. A woman's bone density peaks at about the age of 35, thereafter it reduces at approximately 1 per cent a year.

The bone density and its rate of decrease is highly variable and one of the main factors is the amount of weight-bearing exercise the person does.

Bone is a living tissue, it varies in structure according to the workload expected of it and the type of forces transmitted through it. In short, the more active weight-bearing exercise that a person can do, the greater their bone mass will be, their bone density loss will be reduced, and they will have a much lower risk of developing osteoporosis. Sitting, with its complete absence of weight-bearing exercise must be regarded as an important osteoporosis risk factor. Get off that seat and exercise as often as possible! If you have to sit a lot make sure you have an active exercise programme by way of compensation. Good nutrition with adequate levels of calcium is also important.

OBESITY

Sitting uses very few calories. It is entirely inactive. For people who sit a majority of the day, this can be a factor in promoting obesity and its associated health risks such as heart disease and arthritis.

There are two ways to combat this.

- An active exercise programme.
- Sensible nutrition.

In the section on circulation we discussed the difficulties of getting an adequate blood supply to the brain. One of the consequences of an inadequate supply of blood is a drop in energy provision to the nervous system. There is a natural tendency to compensate for this by eating energy-rich foods. This explains the desire to snack and the popularity of morning and afternoon teas. These snacks are usually high in calories and can contribute to the general problem of ingesting more calories than we are able to use up. Once again exercise and movement will help supply the brain with its essential energy requirements by improving the blood supply. Snacks and diet generally should be based on low-calorie and high-roughage foods such as fruit, salads, wholegrain products with low sugar and fat content. More detailed dietary advice for the sedentary worker is given in chapter 10.

SUMMARY

The lack of exercise produced by sitting can have a detrimental effect on health. It can cause:

- Circulatory problems and their complications, such as heart disease and venous thrombosis.
- Osteoporosis.
- Obesity.

The sitting posture can cramp the abdomen and thorax, affecting the quality of digestion and breathing.

These health effects can be compensated for by regular exercise, good dietary management and paying careful attention to posture.

3

Is sitting bad for your back?

THE UPRIGHT SPINE

The human spine is perfectly developed for the normal standing posture. In this position it has strength, good mobility and is well balanced. It requires a minimum of muscular effort to maintain this position and can do so with relatively little strain.

The spine consists of a series of curves. It has been estimated that these curves lead to an increase in strength which is 10 times greater than that of a straight column. Each curve is designed for a different function, and its structure reflects this.

The cervical (neck) curve has seven relatively small vertebrae (spinal bones). They are designed to allow good movement, but not to transmit large amounts of weight or force. Most of the rotation comes from the upper cervical spine and most of the forward and backward bending from the lower cervical spine.

The thoracic curve is designed to carry an intermediate

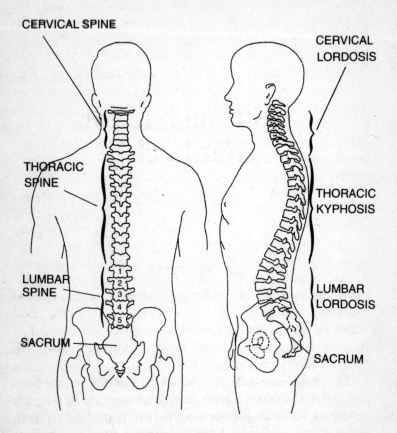

Fig. 3.1a The spinal column
when standing – rear view.

Fig. 3.1b The spinal column
when standing – side view.

amount of weight and force, and is a relatively inflexible part of the spine. Its mobility is affected by the rib cage; there is a rib attached to each side of the 12 thoracic vertebrae.

The lumbar spine is built for strength. There are five big strong vertebrae designed to absorb forces and transmit weight. It is quite mobile in forward and backward bending, but has less side bending and rotation.

The cervical and lumbar curves follow the same direction, known as a lordosis. The thoracic curve follows the opposite direction, known as a kyphosis.

At the base of the spine is the sacrum. This is a triangular block of bone which consists of five vertebrae joined together. At the tip of the sacrum is the coccyx which is all that remains of a tail we once had. The sacrum fits snugly between the two pelvic bones with two large strong joints known as the sacroiliac joints. These transmit the weight and force through to the pelvis and have only a small amount of movement.

The hip joints are very strong ball and socket joints. Like most stable joints they have strong muscles and ligaments. They transmit the force from the pelvis to the lower limbs.

The front portion of each vertebra is designed for strength. It has a large strong vertebral body. These become larger and stronger as they progress down the spine. Between the vertebral bodies are the discs. These are very cleverly designed to absorb forces and at the same time allow some rocking movement between each segment. They have a tough rubbery outside made of cartilage known as the annulus, and a semi-fluid, jelly-like centre known as the nucleus.

The spinal cord runs down the centre of the vertebral column, just behind the vertebral bodies. One of the main functions of the spine is to protect the spinal cord. Just

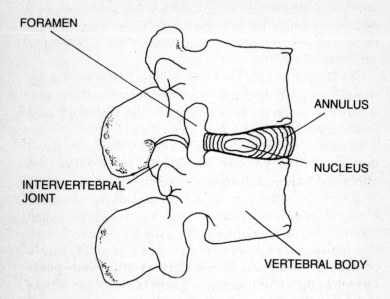

Fig. 3.2 The vertebral unit.

behind the disc there is a hole either side of the vertebra
called a foramen. From these foramina nerve roots leave
the spinal cord and travel to various parts of the body. This
is a very common area for trapped nerves such as in sciatica
when the nerve leaving the spinal cord is trapped at the
level of the fourth or fifth lumbar vertebra.

Just behind the foramina on either side of the spine are
the intervertebral joints. It is the shape and angle of these
joints that determine the type of movement at each level.
Between each level there are a total of three joints: the disc,
and the two intervertebral joints. These form a stable
tripod arrangement. Movement at any one joint will

automatically affect the other two joints. This can make diagnosis of spinal problems very tricky, as movement in a particular area of the spine will influence a number of structures simultaneously.

Muscles are required to move joints, and ligaments act as stabilisers to restrict the movement at a joint. The vertebra has three projections that provide attachments for the ligaments and muscles in positions that enhance their leverage. There is one either side known as the lateral process, and one at the back known as the spinous process. You can see the tips of the spinous processes when looking at a person's back.

THE SITTING SPINE

When we sit down the normal shape of our spine changes. This has a major effect on the way the joints work and the types of stresses they are exposed to.

In an unsupported sitting position, the spine, instead of having a series of three curves, now only has one long curve. This one long curve only has twice the strength of a straight column (as opposed to 10 times the strength with the three curves). The more exaggerated this curve becomes the weaker it is.

In the sitting position, the lumbar curve completely reverses, the thoracic curve increases, becoming more kyphotic, and the cervical curve tends to reverse, depending on head position. These changes in position of the vertebrae also affect the soft tissues around the spine. The ligaments at the back of the spine stretch, while the ligaments at the front of the spine, the inside of the curve, slacken. The muscles at the back of the spine stretch and tend to work harder to prevent the spine falling further into the curve, while the muscles in front of the spine relax and

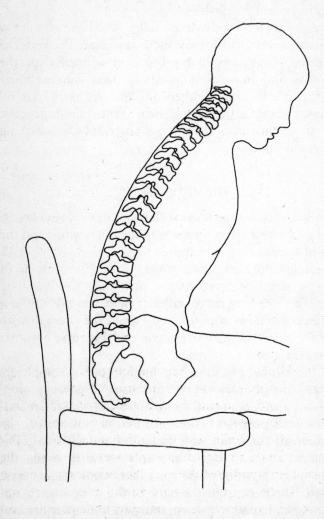

Fig. 3.3 The shape of the spine when sitting.

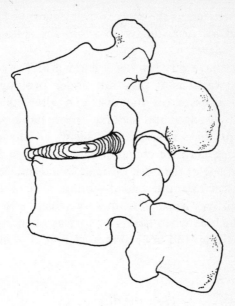

Fig. 3.4 The vertebral unit when sitting. Note the compression and bulging of the disc.

tend to weaken. The discs become squashed and distorted as they attempt to absorb the extra forces.

Muscles and ligaments are richly endowed with sensory nerves. If they are stressed for any period of time they send messages to the brain which manifest as aches or pains. When we start to feel discomfort we alter our sitting posture to try and give some of these tissues a period of rest. If we sit too long, or are forced into a particular posture for a long period, we can start to damage our soft tissues. It usually starts with muscle fatigue, then strain, and ultimately produces injury. We must learn to listen to our bodies giving us the early warning signs of fatigue and strain, and act accordingly to avoid the serious injuries before they develop.

The discs have very few nerve endings and as a result are unable to warn us if they are under prolonged stress. Prolonged stresses on the disc can alter its structure, reducing its strength and making it more liable to injury. It can also produce a premature ageing of the disc, with resulting degenerative changes. The long-term disc problem can be one of the most difficult spinal injuries to treat. It can be very painful and disabling, and even when it finally improves it can remain very sensitive to increased pressure such as when sitting or forward bending. With a little knowledge and understanding these disc injuries can be avoided.

How the disc works

The disc is the main cushion between the vertebrae. It has an amazing capacity to absorb shock, and at the same time be able to change shape and allow spinal flexibility.

The outside of the disc, the annulus, has rows of fibrous tissue, running obliquely to each other. These have some properties of elasticity, so that they can stretch and return to normal. They function as ligaments, so that whichever way the joint is moved there will always be some fibres that prevent excessive movement. They have an important role in maintaining a constant internal pressure. This internal pressure is necessary to prevent the disc collapsing under normal loads.

The annulus is very effective in retaining the semi-fluid nucleus within the disc. Occasionally the nucleus can leak out, but it requires a degeneration of the annulus for this to

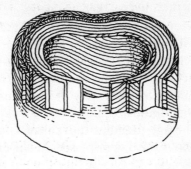

Fig. 3.5 The structure of the annulus.

happen. Leakage of the disc nucleus is known as a prolapsed disc and is very painful and slow healing, as the fluid usually interferes with the nerve roots that form the sciatic nerve. Fortunately this is not a common cause of back pain, but when it occurs it is one of the most difficult problems to treat. The so-called 'slipped disc' is a misnomer, and not an accurate description of what happens when a disc is damaged. The nucleus of the disc is a jellylike, semi-fluid substance containing complex chemicals which help maintain the internal pressure in the disc. The nucleus contains water, cartilage and a number of different types of cells. These cells require an exchange of fluid in the disc to provide their nutrition and remove their waste products. The discs do not have a normal arterial blood supply, as the internal pressure would disrupt it. The cells receive their fluid supply by a process of diffusion from the vertebral body through to the disc. The chemicals in the nucleus are able to attract fluid to them, which helps maintain the internal pressure. If the pressure on the disc increases some of the fluid is squeezed out, and if the disc pressure reduces fluid is sucked in again. It is this fluid exchange, between the vertebral body and the disc, which provides the nutrition essential to the health of the disc. When we are lying down at night and the disc pressure is low the disc sucks in fluid and increases the height of the disc. Throughout the working day the pressure on the disc can produce a net outflow of fluid, and we can lose height by the disc shrinkage. Regular movement and changes of posture throughout the day are essential for optimum disc health and efficiency.

Prolonged pressure on the disc tends to force out the fluid and deforms the annulus rendering the disc less effective as a shock absorber. This causes the disc to become squashed. It is this prolonged pressure that reduces the nutrition available to the disc, bulges the annulus and contributes to a gradual deterioration and an increased susceptibility to injury. After a period of continuous pressure the disc is going to be significantly less effective if asked to cope with a sudden load. Lifting a suitcase out of the boot might normally be quite straightforward, but at the end of a long car journey when the spine has been under continuous pressure it could be a very risky thing to do. In this situation the disc requires a recovery period, before it is able to function efficiently.

> A healthy disc requires regular movement and the avoidance of prolonged forward bent postures, such as sitting and bending. So don't watch too much television; walk instead of ride; use the stairs rather than the lift; if you have to sit, have regular activity breaks. KEEP ACTIVE!

Disc pressure

There are times when it is necessary to sit, and it is a feature of modern life that there is an ever-increasing trend towards more sitting, whether for work, relaxation or travel. We've established how the greater the pressure on the disc the more difficult it is for the disc to function effectively and the more likely it is for the disc to deteriorate and become injured. When we sit we need to choose the sitting postures that have the least disc pressure. As a general principle the more erect the spine is, the closer it is to a normal standing posture and the lower the pressure in the disc.

During standing the weight on each vertebra is shared between the disc and the intervertebral joints. Any forward-bending movement places additional pressure on the disc while reducing it on the intervertebral joints. Any disc pressure greater than that of standing erect tends to squeeze fluid out of the discs.

Most chairs have some kind of back support, and it has been shown that the position of the back support and the angle of the trunk can make a significant difference to the disc pressure. It has also been established that extra lumbar support and the use of arm rests can reduce disc pressure. Obviously this only applies if the back rest and arm rest are used. They provide no benefit whatsoever if a person has to lean forward to work over a horizontal desk.

Sitting tends to be a dynamic activity. People assume different sitting postures for different jobs and constantly like to alter their postures. This is beneficial, and if there is sufficient variation it will benefit disc nutrition. Therefore seating has to be designed to allow a variety of postures.

The disc pressure that is generated by bending and lifting a weight from the ground is far larger than that created by sitting. The danger of the disc pressure generated by sitting is that it lasts much longer and that we do it for a greater proportion of the day.

DISC PRESSURES

Posture	Pressure (%)
Lifting 20kg: knees straight	485
knees bent	265
Sitting forward bent	180
Sitting typing	175
Standing, leaning forward 20°	170
Writing at desk	145
Sitting slumped	140
Sitting up straight	125
Leaning on back rest of office chair	120
STANDING	100
Lying on side	75
Sitting reclined: 20° back rest	75
40° back rest	55
Lying on back	35

Adapted from Pheasant (1991). Data from Nachemson and Elfström (1979); Andersson and Ortengren (1974); Andersson et al. (1974).

There is no available data for disc pressure on forward tilt chairs. I would expect it to be somewhere between standing (100) and sitting upright (125).

> For good spinal health make sure your sitting posture
> has as low a disc pressure as possible (close to 100 per
> cent on the table).
> Make sure you have frequent postural changes,
> including standing and walking.

Disc injuries

It is not the purpose of this book to discuss the diagnosis
and treatment of back problems. However, I would like to
explain a little more about the problems that can afflict the
intervertebral disc, because I believe that the extra pressure
caused by sitting is a major factor in disc injuries.

Just as every tissue in our body ages, the intervertebral
discs show characteristic changes with passing time. The
semi-fluid nucleus shows a gradual dehydration, becoming
firmer. It is gradually replaced with a network of fibrous
tissue which becomes less distinguishable from the annulus. The annulus also dehydrates and shows a gradual
reduction in elasticity. These changes cause a reduction in
height of the disc (the reason why people can gradually
shrink with age) and a stiffening of the spine.

These changes seem to be protective in the long term.
They increase stability and prevent the extreme postures
that cause stress to the spine. The peak incidence of back
problems is 35 to 40 years, with a significant reduction
over the age of 50 after the spine has begun to stiffen.

Extra stress on the vertebrae can show a premature
ageing of the disc and the intervertebral joints. The point at
which normal ageing becomes premature degenerative
change is very difficult to define. Industrial injury tribunals
all over the world grapple with this tricky problem. It can

be clearly shown on x-ray or more modern imaging techniques such as ultra sound scan, that different discs deteriorate at different rates. One disc may show advanced degenerative changes while its neighbour might be in relatively fine fettle.

Disc degenerative change itself does not cause pain. As we noted earlier, there are no nerve endings inside the disc capable of transmitting pain. The problem that arises with disc degenerative change is that the disc becomes a less effective shock absorber and can easily be injured when subjected to more force than it can cope with.

A normal disc under normal strains will not cause pain. An abnormal disc under the common strains of sitting can become troublesome even though it may not have given any previous signs of its premature degenerative change. The most common sites for disc injury are the two lowest discs in the lumbar spine which bear the most weight and are subject to considerable forces.

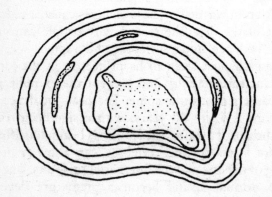

Fig. 3.6 The bulging intervertebral disc.

The problems arise when the concentric layers of the annulus start to deteriorate with the continued pressure. The constant bulging they are subjected to weakens their structure and increases the internal pressure further. It is this bulging that can cause pressure on the sensitive tissues around the nerve roots and the spinal cord and can cause an aching or burning pain which is aggravated by sitting and bending. There can often be referred pain into the buttocks or legs and sometimes a full sciatica. At this stage the problem is reversible. Alleviation of the pressure will give the disc a chance to recover, and with sensible management and treatment the pain will ease, though the disc may remain sensitive to further pressure.

If the pressure is continued the disc injury may progress to the next and more serious stage, the disc prolapse. As the annulus bulges and weakens, fissures start to appear in the fibres. The increasing disc pressure starts to force the semi-fluid nucleus through these fissures which can initially

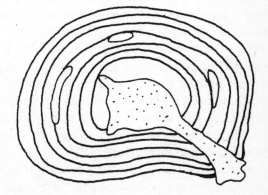

Fig. 3.7 The prolapsed intervertebral disc.

aggravate the bulging disc but can eventually burst through the annular wall. This is nasty. It usually causes pressure in the narrow canals where the spinal nerves exit. The extrusion of the nucleus sets up an inflammatory reaction in this small space and the result can be excruciating nerve pain, numbness and muscle weakness, such as exists with sciatica. It can take a long time for the body to break down this extruded nucleus and the recovery is measured over months rather than weeks. With good care and patience, surgery is not usually necessary.

The vulnerable age for disc injuries is when the annulus starts to deteriorate with extra pressure, but the nucleus is not sufficiently dehydrated to lose its fluidity and is able to be squeezed out; a bit like toothpaste from a tube. The danger period is probably between 30 and 40 years of age.

The good news is that this nasty problem can be avoided. Good posture and sensible management avoid the excess pressure that creates the premature degeneration in the disc and avoid the forces responsible for the disc bulge and subsequent prolapse. If you can understand this important principle you can protect yourself against disc injuries.

As the disc compresses and degenerates and the annulus shows an increased bulging, the bony vertebral bodies try to adapt to this. The adaptation involves the formation of bony spurs at the vertebral body margins to try and reinforce the bulging disc. When these are seen on x-ray they signify that the vertebral disc and joints have advanced degenerative changes. While this is not painful, it does suggest that this segment is weak and prone to injury if stressed by extra weight or pressure.

The narrowing of the disc also causes an increased pressure in the intervertebral joints and these respond by producing bony extensions at the edges of the inter-vertebral joints. These bony spurs, or osteophytes, can

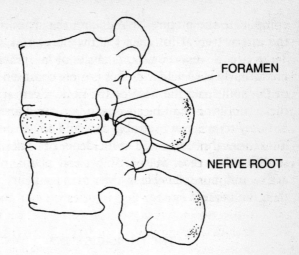

FORAMEN

NERVE ROOT

Fig. 3.8a The healthy spinal segment.

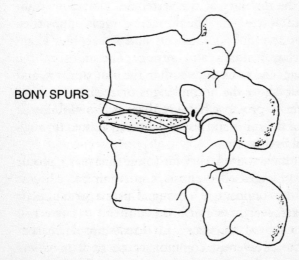

BONY SPURS

Fig. 3.8b The degenerative spinal segment. Note the thinning of the disc, and the bony spurs encroaching on the foramen.

complicate the picture by reducing the space available in the intervertebral foramen for the nerve root to emerge. They are a very common cause of a 'pinched nerve' particularly in the elderly. This is most common at the base of the spine and the base of the neck. Even at this stage, these conditions can be successfully treated and managed, but they require very sensible care and an awareness of the limitations they impose. The incidence of back pain decreases after the age of 50, partly because people become less active and more sensible in their management. They know their limitations.

THE THORACIC SPINE

The thoracic spine extends from the base of the neck to the bottom of the rib cage. Each of the twelve thoracic vertebra has a rib attached to either side and the structure of the rib cage limits the mobility of the vertebrae, providing additional structural strength. The thoracic curve is opposite to the lumbar curve; it is a kyphosis and it becomes exaggerated during bending and sitting. The discs in the thoracic spine tend to be thinner than the lumbar discs, and while they do show the normal signs of ageing it is quite rare for them to prolapse because there is less mobility in this region of the spine and less weight transmitted through the vertebral bodies.

You don't have to look very far to see that many people suffer from an increased kyphosis, commonly described as round shoulders or dowager's hump. This is a form of poor posture that once it is established is difficult to correct. It can be caused by osteoporosis in elderly people, particularly women. The most common cause of it in young people is too much sitting in poor postures while they go through the rapid growth phase of adolescence.

SCHEUERMANN'S DISEASE (SD)

This is the name given to a condition involving degenerative changes of the spine which affects teenagers. It is extraordinarily common. One study in New Zealand of 500 teenagers (Fisk et al., 1984) showed that 56 per cent of males and 30 per cent of females had x-ray evidence of the presence of SD.

It could well be that a significant proportion of the readers of this book had SD during their youth. A previous history of SD significantly increases the risk of developing back pain later in life, and one study showed that it more than doubles the incidence of disc degenerative disease in the lumbar spine (Stoddard and Osborn, 1979).

It is worthwhile going into a little detail about the cause and development of SD, because with a little understanding it can be avoided. For those people who may have already had the condition (the changes are permanent), understanding the nature of the condition may help them avoid some of the possible complications. It occurs between the ages of 11 and 17, usually becoming active for about 12 months. It is associated with a growth spurt and what appears to be a relative osteoporosis as the bones grow too fast and become temporarily weakened. It commonly affects two or more vertebrae between the seventh thoracic and the first lumbar vertebrae.

The increased compression from prolonged sitting on the weakened vertebral bodies of the thoracic spine leads to a characteristic deformity. The young healthy discs are better able to withstand this pressure, and it is the vertebral bodies that deform under the pressure showing irregularities at the edges and the characteristic wedging of an increased kyphosis.

The Fisk study showed that there were a number of

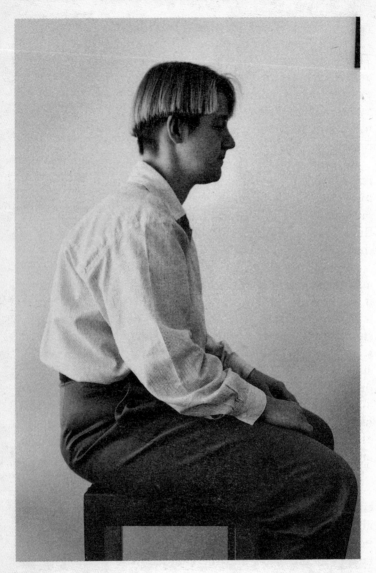

Fig. 3.9 Poor sitting position can lead to permanent change in posture. Note the increased thoracic and cervical curves.

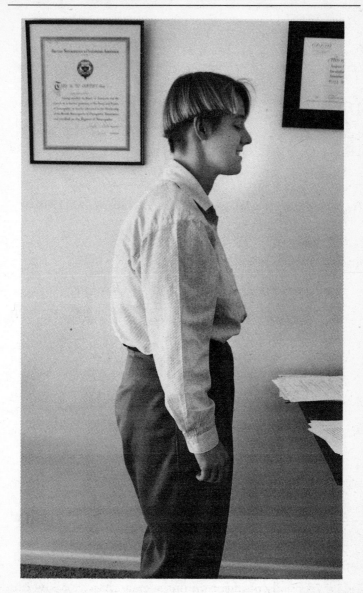

Fig. 3.10 Note the standing posture.

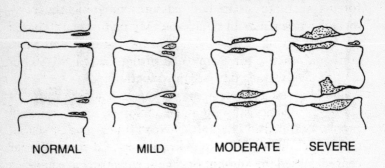

NORMAL   MILD   MODERATE   SEVERE

Fig. 3.11 The effect of Scheuermann's disease. (Adapted from Fisk 1987).

factors relating to the presence of SD.

- Long periods of bed rest caused an increased incidence. The bone structure was probably weakened through lack of exercise.
- Over half reported a history of back pain lasting more than one week. It does not necessarily cause pain during the active phase.
- There was a relationship between tight hamstrings and SD.
- There was an increased incidence in people with an exaggerated kyphosis.
- There were characteristic muscular changes over the thoracic spine. Dr J. Fisk states: 'The paravertebral muscles had a ropey quality, probably signifying prolonged increased activity, and they were irritable and more tender than it was felt they should be.'
- Tall males were more prone to severe SD.

It is a very sad comment on our society that we allow our young people to do themselves such significant damage by forcing them to sit in bad postures pursuing the ever-increasing demands of education. My own research based on interviewing school children has shown that it is common practice for them to be sitting for at least 80 per cent of their waking day (see introduction).

The amount of time spent sitting is a major cause of spinal problems in school-age children. In a research project outlined in chapter 7, over 90 per cent of school children complained of spinal problems. Of these, 71 per cent identified the amount of time spent sitting at school as a major factor.

I am continually dismayed that more attention is not paid to designing and providing our youth with good furniture that allows correct posture and minimises the incidence of SD and related spinal problems. Good posture means being able to sit up straight to work at a high sloping desk, rather than hunching over a low horizontal desk. There are some measures that we can take to try and prevent our children developing this condition.

- A good-quality, well-designed desk and chair for home-work and study.
- An active sport or exercise programme to strengthen the spine and muscles.
- Stretching exercises to ensure good spinal mobility and to stretch the tight hamstring muscles.
- Good nutrition (especially calcium).
- Turn off the TV, video and computer! At least try and restrict the amount of sitting for leisure.

These same measures will assist the adult who may have the changes of SD present in their adult form and who wishes to avoid the possible complications. It can be seen that the genesis of disc degenerative change and Scheuermann's disease are very closely related, and the methods of avoiding these problems and their complications are very similar. The changes of old SD tend to produce a characteristically stiff segment of the spine with tight ropey muscles and very tight hamstrings. It is a mechanically inefficient spine that is prone to further injury.

THE CERVICAL SPINE

The part of the spine that forms the neck. It has seven small vertebrae which do not have to transmit large amounts of weight. They are very mobile, allowing us a good field of vision. They are very prone to injury by external force, such as a whiplash or head injury.

There don't seem to be many people who haven't had a neck injury at some time in their lives. The neck is very happy to hold the head up in an erect position where it is well balanced, but it very soon tires of holding the head at one of its extremes of motion. The main problem with sitting is usually holding the head forward to work at a horizontal surface, such as a desk or table. This dramatically increases the pressure in the lower cervical discs and makes the small neck muscles work very hard. The early effects of this are neck tension, neck stiffness and headaches, but in the long term this can lead to disc and joint degenerative change in the lower cervical vertebrae. The degeneration of the cervical vertebrae occurs in much the same way as that of the lumbar vertebrae as described earlier. The increased mobility in the neck, the habitual poor postures we adopt and the high injury rate of the cervical spine result in the lower neck being the most common site in the spine for degenerative changes. Once these degenerative changes have begun, the cervical spine suffers a decreased tolerance to the stresses and strains of

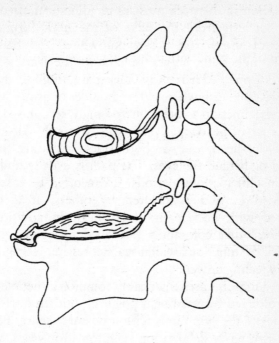

Fig. 3.12 Degenerative change in the cervical spine.

awkward or prolonged postures and becomes more suscep-
tible to further strain and injury. An awareness of the
problem, combined with effective management, means that
the degenerative problems need not cause pain and other
associated symptoms. Understanding the principles of
good posture, a well-designed work environment and
effective work management skills can help avoid the build
up of these conditions.

The muscles in the neck usually give us early warning if
they are overworked, and if you have neck stiffness, neck
pain or headaches, this is an indication that all is not well.

Inflammation in the neck muscles or joints can affect the nerves that exit from the base of the neck forming a network of interlacing nerves known as the brachial plexus. From here the nerves travel down the arms, and an inflamed or pinched nerve can cause pain, tingling, numbness or weakness anywhere in the shoulder or arm.

Neck dysfunction is being increasingly recognised as a major cause of headaches. The pain is usually felt at the back of the head, one or both sides, radiating to the forehead or behind the eyes. The pain is usually dull and quite constant for long periods. It can often be eased by some postures and aggravated by others. It is often associated with neck pain or stiffness. In addition to headaches, other commonly described problems arising from neck dysfunction are: nausea, depression, vertigo and generally feeling unwell.

These symptoms are remarkably common in people who sit in prolonged forward bent postures, but they often do not associate the symptoms with a postural cause. People put up with nasty debilitating symptoms for years, when the solutions are quite simple and can often be easily remedied.

4

Oh my aching muscles!

Muscles give us the power of movement. They enable us to move all or part of our bodies and hold them in different positions. Without the use of muscles we would be unable to maintain a standing or sitting posture.

Each muscle consists of thousands of muscle fibres. The muscle fibres are bound together into bundles called fasciculi. Each muscle fibre is surrounded by connective tissue. This joins onto the connective tissue that surrounds each fasciculus. The connective tissue that surrounds each fasciculus is contiguous with the connective tissues enveloping the muscle. This network of connective tissue joins together at either end of the muscle to form the tendons. The tendon attaches the muscle to the bone. Tendons can have a localised attachment, or they can have a more expansive attachment.

Each muscle fibre has the ability to contract – it is able to shrink to half its length. The longer a muscle is when it begins its contraction, the more power is available for the contraction. This is one of the reasons we recommend stretching exercises. A shortened, stiffened muscle is less

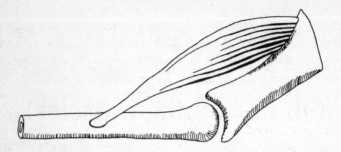

Fig. 4.1 The structure of muscle. Note the bundles of muscle fibres and the continuous connective tissue that surrounds them.

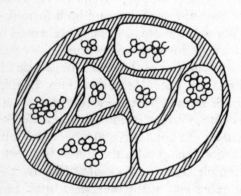

Fig. 4.2 Cross-section of a muscle.

efficient than one able to stretch to its full length.

The muscle is connected to the brain by nerves. The motor nerves carry messages from the brain to the muscle telling it when to contract. The nerve splits into fibres, each supplying a number of muscle fibres; the number of nerve fibres that are stimulated determines the power and length of the muscle contraction. In this way the brain is able to fine tune muscle control. Sensory nerves in the muscles provide information to the brain and spinal cord about the amount of tension or stretch in the muscle, which assists in fine tuning the muscle function. Other types of nerve fibres are able to transmit sensations of pain if the muscle becomes fatigued or damaged.

Different muscles have developed a specialised structure that reflects their function. Phasic muscles are strong muscles built to perform rapid movements. They are good for actions that require movement and strength but are not able to sustain this for long without regular breaks. The postural muscles are able to hold sustained positions for longer periods of time, without fatiguing. They are able to do this by different muscle fasciculi contracting in rotation. Postural muscles are usually situated close to a joint and are able to fine tune its position. Although they are able to function for long periods, they do not have the same power as phasic muscles.

A muscle contraction requires energy. This energy comes from chemicals stored in the muscle. In order to continue actively contracting, the muscle has to have fresh supplies of these chemicals. The chemicals require oxygen for the process to release the energy and this process creates waste products, the principal one being lactic acid. If these waste products build up they interfere with the muscle's ability to contract, with resulting pain and stiffness.

The determining factor of how well a muscle can function is the quality of blood supply, providing the factors required for muscle contraction and removal of the waste products.

When a muscle contracts the increased tension shuts off

its blood supply. It requires a period of relaxation to allow the circulation to return. Most methods of movement such as walking and running have a continuous contraction–relaxation muscle action that allows us to continue the action for longer periods of time. This contraction–relaxation cycle acts as a pump squeezing blood out of the muscle during contraction and sucking it in during relaxation. This pumping action is able to increase the blood flow to the muscle by 10 to 20 times.

By contrast a postural muscle or a muscle working in a static position without relaxation is not able to benefit from an increased circulation and will rapidly fatigue if the workload is greater than the ability of the blood supply to sustain it. For this reason I emphasise frequent postural variations when working in a fixed posture such as sitting and regular breaks with change of activity to allow adequate recovery.

MUSCLE STRENGTH

When a muscle works continuously it only has sufficient energy for a short period of time. The stronger the contraction, the shorter the period. Thus:

- Maximum force can be sustained for about one second.
- 70 per cent force can be sustained for about 30 seconds.
- 50 per cent force can be sustained for about one minute.
- 8 per cent force can be sustained for about one hour.

For an eight-hour working day the maximum force able to be sustained seems to be about 3 to 4 per cent of the maximum.

The muscle strength available to a person is subject to predetermined characteristics such as gender and age. There is also a significant lifestyle effect. Regular exercise and use can improve the strength and efficiency of muscle contraction.

Gender

Women tend to have less strength available than men. On average a woman has 60 per cent the strength of a man. This is only an average and can vary markedly between individuals. The average is not constant for all body parts. There tends to be greater gender difference of strength in the upper arms and shoulders and less in the legs.

Age

Maximum strength is reached between the ages of 20 and 25, but remains reasonably constant up to the age of 40 when it starts to decline. By the age of 65 it is approximately 75 per cent of its peak.

Training effects

We do not have much control over our age and gender, and these are factors that can determine our muscle strength and predisposition to injury. However, we do have control over our levels of fitness and the condition of our muscle tissue. Improved muscle conditioning is a major protective factor against overuse injury. Muscle fibres are able to adapt to increased levels of exercise. They do this by increasing the amount of stored chemicals available for muscle contraction and by improving the circulation to the muscle to allow increased transport of oxygen and removal of waste products. So exercise has the following effects:

- It increases the strength of the muscle.
- It improves the stamina of the muscle.
- It speeds up the recovery period.

In addition to these effects, the connective tissue that envelops the muscle fibre and forms the tendons that join the muscle to the bone starts to change in structure and develops the capacity to transmit the increased force. The muscles and tendons do adapt to the work they are required to do but this process of adaptation takes time. It is very easy to overload the muscle and develop an injury somewhere in the muscle–tendon–bone complex when we continuously perform certain tasks. It is therefore wise to start any new activity in graduated stages to allow the tissues to adapt without risking muscle fatigue and injury. The adaptive functions of the muscles and tendons can reverse when we cease the activity. When we return to an activity after a holiday, illness or time away, we need to graduate our resumption of the activity. Usually in these cases the brain has a good memory of the activity – we never forget how to ride a bicycle – but the muscles have lost some of their adaptive properties. It is in these situations where the mind is more willing than the body that the greatest risk of injury lies.

Post-exercise soreness

The stiff and painful muscles that come on after unaccustomed use of a muscle usually develops a few hours after the activity. It peaks on the second day after which it gradually improves. This is a normal response to unaccustomed exercise and will have no lasting effect provided the muscle is allowed to recover fully prior to the activity being repeated.

Muscle overuse

When there is a single muscular workload that causes post-exercise stiffness, the cause and solution are equally obvious. The problems arise when the activity is not sufficient to cause obvious symptoms, but is sufficiently taxing for the muscle to be progressively overloaded. This is commonly found in work situations where an activity does not feel strenuous, but is required to be maintained for an extended period of time. The muscle starts to develop fatigue and physiological changes start to take place in the muscle and its associated soft tissues that reduce its ability to perform efficiently. The muscle starts to become tense and is difficult to relax. It feels ropey and tender to touch. The associated joints start to stiffen.

TRIGGER POINTS (TPs)

The ropey tender points in the muscle are known as trigger points. They are localised areas of muscle fibres that remain in spasm. Active TPs have characteristic findings:

- Localised taut bands, running in the direction of the muscle fibres.
- Tender to touch.
- Pressure on the point is very painful and causes referred pain.
- It often has a twitch response – if you rub gently across it, this can trigger a localised spasm.
- Muscle stiffness.

There is usually more than one TP in a muscle, and careful examination can often reveal a group of them. If the TPs have been present for some time secondary TPs can develop in the area of the referred pain or in other associated muscles. Examination of people who do not have any symptoms often shows the presence of latent TPs. These have the feel of trigger points and are tender to touch, though under normal circumstances they do not cause pain. They remain sensitive and can be easily activated by minor insults such as cold draughts, exercise, minor trauma, etc. They may be the site of previous overuse or trauma that has been successfully deactivated by the healing process.

The TP seems to lose the ability to relax when not in use, maintaining a continual degree of slight muscle contraction with resulting fatigue. The reasons for this are the subject of considerable debate. The changes resulting from fatigue are certainly a factor – lack of oxygen and accumulation of waste products. There also appears to be an overactivity of the nerves that send messages to make the muscle contract. Many people believe that stress is an important precipitating factor in producing the nerve overactivity. In long-standing TPs there is evidence that the body starts to lay down fibrous tissue (scar tissue) throughout the muscle fibres as this has a reduced oxygen requirement.

Once a trigger point has become active there appears to be a self-perpetuating cycle of muscle fatigue–pain–spasm. This reduces the efficiency of the muscle and related joints, increasing the strain that they are subject to. If these inefficiencies are not addressed, and the causative factors remain, the problem progresses with involvement of more trigger points and increased nerve activity.

Trigger point therapy

The aim of therapy is to deactivate the TP, returning the muscle tension to normal and restoring the range of movement to the joint. The methods used to deactivate the TPs are:

- Deep massage techniques.
- Ice, followed by stretching.
- Acupuncture (to the TP sites).
- Muscle stretching exercises.

These principles of treatment have been incorporated in the self-help section of this book on pages 174–231.

The pioneering work on trigger points has been done by two American researchers, Drs Janet Travell and David Simons. Their work, *Myofascial Pain and Dysfunction: The Trigger Point Manual*, volumes 1 and 2 (Williams and Wilkins, 1983 and 1992), is regarded as the classic in its field. The terms 'myofascial pain' and 'trigger point' have largely replaced a host of other confusing terminology such as fibrositis, fibromyositis, myofibrositis, myalgia, etc.

The formation of a TP can arise from a complex interplay of factors, of which the main feature is overuse of the muscle. It is most commonly a cumulative process over a period of time, but can also be secondary to injury or immobilisation. The most consistent factor is overuse of the muscle with inadequate recovery periods. This may be a repetitive use where muscle is continually required to repeat an action, or static use where a muscle is held in sustained tension for long periods without relief. There seems to be a narrow dividing line between where exercise can provide muscle strength and fitness and overuse where it produces the pain–tension–spasm cycle.

It is likely that the continual presence of trigger points and impaired muscle function can lead to problems with the associated joints. These can become progressively stiff with an increased joint pressure, reduced circulation and development of adhesions. If permitted to persist this can lead to postural deformity and an accelerated process of wear and tear, or degeneration of the joint also known as osteoarthritis.

The trigger point theory has developed from the palpable changes associated with fatigued muscle and has developed a method of therapy to relieve this. Its simplicity, its logic and its ready palpability have ensured its popularity with patients and therapists confronted with musculoskeletal problems. Another school of thought has developed to deal with the vexing problem of muscle fatigue. The focus of this approach has come from looking at the cause of the muscle fatigue, rather than the findings in the muscle. Hence the development of the term 'repetitive strain injury'.

REPETITIVE STRAIN INJURY (RSI)

RSI is a term applied to the category of work-related musculoskeletal disorders of the neck, shoulder and arm. It came to prominence in the early 1980s following an epidemic of reported cases in Australia, followed shortly after in other developed countries. It is becoming increasingly recognised as a major cause of pain and disability. Its prevalence is widely linked to the increasing computerisation of the workplace.

The symptoms it describes are not new. Bernardini Ramizinni noted in 1713 when writing about the diseases of scribes and notaries:

The maladies that afflict the clerks aforesaid arise from the three causes: first, constant sitting, secondly the incessant movement of the hand and always in the same direction, thirdly, the strain on the mind from the effort not to disfigure the books.

This is an observant description of what are now regarded as the three principal causes of RSI:

- Fixed posture.
- Repetitive movements.
- Stress.

While in the UK the term RSI has been retained, this is not universal and other terms are also used in other countries.

- Occupational Overuse Syndrome (OOS) – Australia and New Zealand.
- Cumulative Trauma Disorder (CTD) – North America.
- Work Related Upper Limb Disorder (WRULD).
- Occupational Cervicobrachial Disorder (OCD) – Japan.

Causes of RSI

Prolonged or repetitive use of a muscle leads to fatigue. The fatigue process interferes with the blood supply of the muscle, producing a deprivation of oxygen and a build up of waste products. If this overuse and fatigue process persists characteristic changes in the muscle take place, including formation of trigger points and inflammation of the muscle–tendon–bone complex of soft tissues that link the muscle fibres to the bone. This is followed by pro-gressive joint dysfunction and hypersensitivity of the nerve fibres that relate to these structures. It all sounds familiar doesn't it? The physiology of RSI is identical to that of myofascial pain and TPs. The main difference, as I see it, is that the TP school of thought focuses on the changes in muscle as the central theme of its concept, while the RSI school looks to the cause of the initial overuse as its point of reference. Both approaches are equally valid and have much to recommend them. While some of the concepts overlap, the RSI school gives us a perspective to deal with the ergonomics at the workplace, while the TP school gives us a model on which to base our therapeutic approach to the identification and deactivation of trigger points. The most effective results of managing the tricky problem of RSI will come by taking advantage of both schools of thought, whereby we are able to address both the cause of the problem and the symptoms produced.

Types of RSI

RSI is a name given to a category of conditions affecting the neck, shoulder and arm, derived from a common cause. Some of the injuries that fit this category are:

- Rotator cuff strain (shoulder).
- Wrist extensor strain (tennis elbow).
- Wrist flexor strain (golfer's elbow).
- Wrist tendonitis.

Some other terms are used to cover neck and shoulder pain that are less specific:

- Neck shoulder arm syndrome.
- Scapulothoracic pain.
- Tension headache.

These conditions and their management are covered in greater detail in the self-help guide (see pages 174–231).

Stages of RSI

The onset and progression of RSI develops through distinct stages. Sometimes these can take place over a short period with rapid progression to a painful and debilitating injury. More commonly the onset is gradual with a slow progression. It is vital to be aware of and to recognise the early symptoms so that appropriate measures can be taken before it reaches the more advanced stages. It is much easier to manage at stages 1 and 2 than when it is left to 3 and 4 when the secondary complications have begun to develop.

Stage 1

This is characterised by pain anywhere in the arm or upper spine when working in one position for a long period. This could be at work or playing a musical instrument; anything that requires repetitive use while in a fixed posture. The pain disappears promptly when the activity is stopped.

Stage 2

The pain starts to come on early in the activity and might not stop as soon as the activity is curtailed. It starts to become apparent in other non-related activities – peeling vegetables, cleaning, picking up the kettle, etc.

Stage 3

The pain comes on early in the activity and continues long after it has ceased. It starts to interfere with daily life and there are things you try to avoid such as carrying bags or doing household chores. It may start spreading to other muscle groups, often to involve the other arm. It can wake you up at night. The symptoms become more complex, with not just pain but pins and needles, numbness and muscle weakness. Other symptoms such as headaches, depression, dizziness, cold and blue hands can become apparent. You start to think seriously about taking time off work and reducing your activity levels.

Stage 4

Pain is constant and disabling. Work is not possible. The avoidance of pain becomes a dominant factor of life. Sleep can be severely disturbed and is often accompanied by depression and general fatigue. Ordinary tasks become very difficult. The pains are not consistent with new sites occurring and old ones being revisited. The secondary effects of nerve symptoms and circulatory disturbance are a significant feature.

Stages 1 to 3 can usually be successfully treated and managed if the appropriate measures are taken. These include careful analysis of the work station, good work management, regular breaks and appropriate therapy. Stage 4 is very difficult to treat and recovery can be tortuously slow, with little possibility of returning to the type of work that initiated the problem. However, good management and appropriate therapy can improve the quality of life and can lead to a limited return to productive activity.

SUMMARY

The best method of dealing with RSI is prevention, avoiding the poor postures and the repetitive use that characterise the problem. An awareness of the early symptoms is important so that the appropriate changes can be made to stop the condition progressing.

Once RSI is established it requires very careful management including:

- Ergonomic assessment of workplace and posture.
- Good work management with regular breaks.
- Appropriate treatment.
- Self-help – exercises, massage, ice, etc.

MUSCLE IMBALANCE

The act of sitting changes our posture from a balanced series of curves to a shape a bit like a banana. This tends to shorten muscles at the front of our body and to cause generalised and specific muscle weakness to those muscles that are underused in this position.

Sitting causes generalised muscle weakness due to its relative inactivity. Research has shown that people today have less muscle strength and tone than previous generations. This means that their joints have less support from the muscles that envelop and protect them. When they do become active they are more prone to injury. After the first fine weekend of spring, my clinic is always full of patients who have injured themselves through overactivity – gardening, tennis, etc., after a winter of inactivity.

I encourage people who sit a lot to take up some form of regular exercise to counteract the weakening effects of their

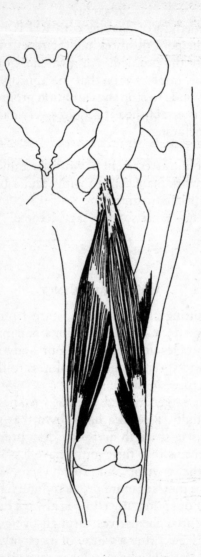

Fig. 4.3 The hamstring muscles.

sedentary lifestyles. Starting a new kind of activity is a time when the soft tissues are easily overstrained before they have a chance to adapt and so particular care is needed. Advice on beginning an exercise programme is covered in chapter 10.

Hamstring muscles

The hamstrings are a group of three muscles at the back of the thigh. They run from the base of the pelvis across the hip and the knee joints inserting just below the knee. They are strong muscles, important for helping to maintain an upright posture, and are involved in all movements of the hip and knee.

The sitting position shortens and weakens these muscles.

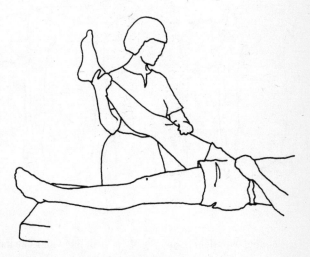

Fig. 4.4 Testing for hamstring tightness.

Tight hamstrings are a very common finding. They usually begin to tighten when children start school at the age of five or six, and deteriorate by the time they reach secondary school.

Studies have shown a link between tight hamstrings and low-back problems. In particular there seems to be a relationship between tight hamstrings and Scheuermann's disease (see pages 41–6).

It is quite easy to check if you have tight hamstrings. They are best tested with the help of a friend. Lie on your back on a flat surface, then ask your friend to raise one of your legs slowly holding it just underneath the heel. Make sure your leg is straight and relaxed. Keep lifting the leg

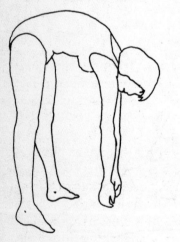

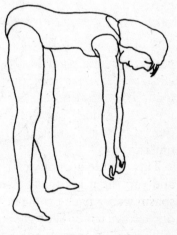

Fig. 4.5a Bending with tight hamstrings.

Fig. 4.5b Bending with loose hamstrings enables you to keep a straight back.

until you feel the tightness in the back of the leg together with an increased resistance. Don't force it further than this otherwise it will twist the pelvis and distort the result of your test.

If the tightness comes on at less than 45° this is regarded as being very tight; 45–60° – moderately tight; 60–75° – could be better; 75° and over – good. Hamstring stretching exercises are shown in chapter 9. People who are active in sports have a lower incidence of hamstring tightness.

Tight hamstrings tend to reduce the amount of bending available in the hip and pelvis. This puts a lot of stress on the low-back during bending and lifting, and it may be one of the reasons for the link between tight hamstrings and low-back problems. Loose hamstrings enable you to keep a nice straight back when bending. Both hamstrings should stretch equally. This is important for good pelvic balance.

Iliopsoas muscles

This is a group of muscles that arise from the spine and pelvis, crossing over the front of the lumbar spine, pelvic and hip joints, inserting into the inside of the thigh. Their main role is to bend the trunk at the hips or to pull the hip up to the trunk. They also help to keep a lumbar curve during bending and lifting. They are important postural muscles.

This muscle group is markedly shortened during sitting and can often gradually tighten. It can go into a painful spasm with a back problem. When this muscle is shortened or spasmed it is difficult to stand up straight after sitting. If it is in spasm on one side only it tends to pull the trunk forward and to the same side. The stooped posture of a psoas spasm is quite easy to recognise. It can sometimes go into spasm with acute abdominal problems such as appendicitis.

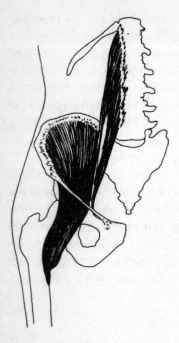

Fig. 4.6 The iliopsoas muscles.

Fig. 4.7 Testing for iliopsoas tightness.

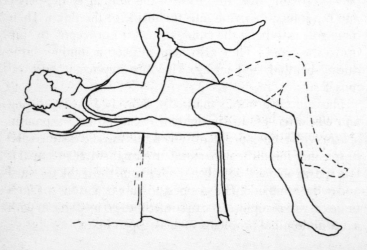

There is a simple test for iliopsoas tightness. Lie on your back on a firm bed with your legs hanging over the end. Hug one knee firmly toward the chest and allow the other leg to drop down. If the iliopsoas is tight the leg will fail to drop below the horizontal. If it drops below the horizontal it is normal. Stretches for the iliopsoas muscles are in chapter 9.

Abdominal muscles

The abdominal muscles are not postural muscles; they are not actively required to contract to maintain normal posture. They are important movers of the trunk however. The rectus abdominis is a strong flexor of the trunk and the oblique abdominal muscles are involved in bending and twisting movements of the trunk.

When we sit the stomach muscles completely relax – you can feel their looseness. Their opposing muscles, the spinal extensors, have to work very hard in this position and this can lead to an imbalance between these two muscle groups. Good muscle tone is very important protection for the spine. There are three reasons for this:

- Good stomach muscle tone counteracts the pull of the spinal extensors. Weak stomach muscle tone can lead to an exaggeration of the normal lumbar curve causing a sway back and placing extra stress on the spinal joints and their ligaments.
- Contraction of the stomach muscles increases the abdominal pressure. In forward bend positions the abdomen then acts as a cushion which takes a lot of unnecessary stress off the spine. Taking a deep breath and contracting the stomach muscles during a lifting movement can reduce the stress on the spine and the

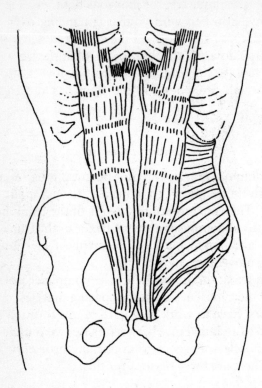

Fig. 4.8a The rectus and transverse abdominal muscles.

work performed by the spinal muscles by 50 per cent,
providing you have good stomach muscle tone.
• The stomach muscles attach to the lumbar fascia and
  spinal vertebrae by a series of guy rope-like attachments which act to strengthen and stabilise the spine.

Good stomach muscle tone is very important protection for

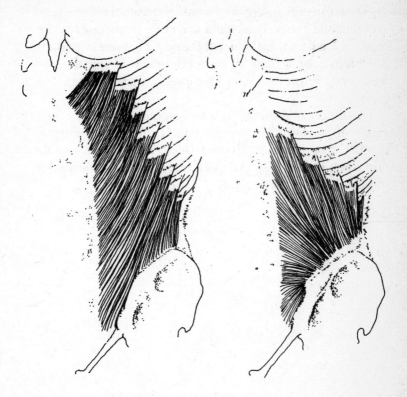

Fig. 4.8b The oblique abdominal muscles.

the spine. The easiest way to test your stomach muscle tone is by trying the abdominal curl exercises in chapter 9.

Another common giveaway is a generalised sagging appearance of the abdomen! Correct abdominal breathing aids good muscle tone.

Summary

Tight hamstring muscles and weak abdominal muscle tone are epidemic in our society and will be an important feature in anyone who sits for much of the day. They are important predetermining factors in the development of spinal problems and, if present, can continually aggravate an old injury.

The iliopsoas muscles tend to become problematic as a result of injury. They can be painful and affect normal posture if they become dysfunctional. They are an important cause of low-back pain as a result of sitting, making it difficult to stand up straight.

5

Sensible sitting

The type of sitting posture we adopt depends on the environment in which we are sitting. The positioning of the lower back is largely determined by the type of chair we are sitting on. The position of the upper spine is mainly decided by our visual needs – positioning our eyes where we can effectively view the task at hand. The position of our shoulders and arms is determined by the task required of them and the arrangement of the equipment for that task. The legs are usually positioned so they can be conveniently placed on the floor to assist with balance and stability. So our posture is largely dependent on:

- The seat.
- The task at hand.
- The arrangement of equipment to perform the task.
- Individual preference.

JOINT COMFORT ZONE

There are some postures that are considerably less stressful to the body than others, and this chapter will outline some of the general principles for the most comfortable sitting positions. Each joint has a position where it is balanced – where the muscle and soft tissues around the joint are functioning in a way that does not overstress them. The further it moves away from this position the more likely it is to develop strain. This is known as the joint comfort zone and our body works most efficiently when we keep our joints within this zone. The joint comfort zone is generally within the middle one third of the range of joint movement.

JOINT COMFORT ZONE

The position of a joint where it works at optimum efficiency with the minimum amount of strain.

It is important when choosing a good sitting posture to ensure that your joints are kept within their comfort zone.

POSTURAL VARIATION

It is not desirable to find an ideal posture and maintain it continuously. It is advisable to vary the posture at regular intervals; to alternate the tissues of the body that are under stress at any particular time.

Sitting should be a dynamic activity with frequent movement of the body parts. This is helpful for the following reasons:

- To relieve any pressure points.
- To prevent build up of excess heat and perspiration.

- To prevent overstress of muscles and ligaments.
- To enhance the circulation – particularly to the inter-vertebral discs.

Postures within the joint comfort zones are generally able to be held with comfort for longer than postures outside the zone.

THE IDEALISED SITTING POSITION

Experts from all over the world have generally considered that the upright sitting position, consisting of a series of right angles, is the correct one. One can see the appeal – it is neat and tidy and looks good on paper. This has become

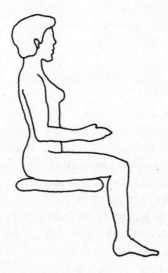

Fig. 5.1 The idealised sitting position.

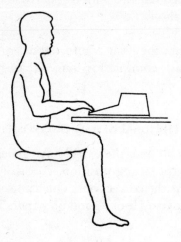

Fig. 5.2 Sitting posture as recommended by a guide to good sitting.

the standard on which furniture manufacturers have based their designs.

In reality it is impossible to hold this posture for more than a few minutes. It requires a considerable amount of muscular effort and strain, and it becomes difficult to perform a task while maintaining this position. Despite this, it continues to be recommended as an example of good sitting posture by most influential authorities.

I continue to be surprised that despite ample evidence of the problems associated with this type of posture, it continues to be widely recommended. The right-angled posture is based on a false assumption. It assumes that when moving from a standing to a sitting position the hip

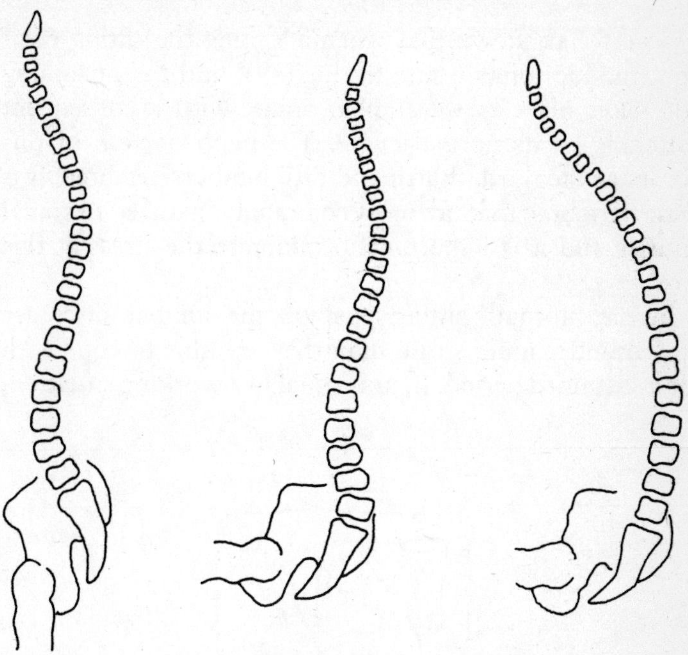

Fig. 5.3 The shape of the spine.
(a)   Standing posture.
(b)   Idealised sitting posture.
(c)   The real sitting posture.

joint flexes to 90°, but the spinal posture remains the same. This is a fallacy. Let's have a closer look at what happens to the spine and pelvis when we sit.

Lumbar spine, pelvis and hips

Research has shown that when adopting the sitting position, the hip joints rotate through 60° and the remaining 30° takes place in the lumbar spine, with a consequent flattening of its normal curve. The main portion of this occurs at the third, fourth and fifth lumbar vertebrae. It is these vertebrae that are most commonly involved in spinal injuries and it is important to minimise the stress at this level.

In the 'normal' sitting position the lumbar discs are placed under more strain than they are able to cope with for a sustained period. If, as is usual in a working situation,

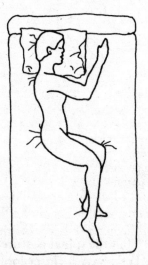

Fig. 5.4 The most common sleeping position, with the hips in a relaxed position.

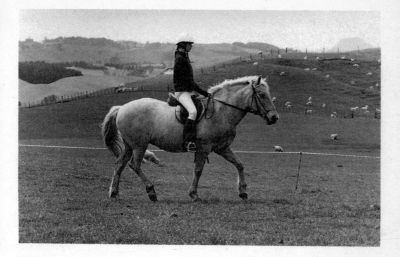

Fig. 5.5 The horse riding posture, an example of good spinal balance.

the body is required to lean forward for reading or writing, the pressure in the lumbar discs increases considerably. The result is increased strain in the lumbar discs and spinal ligaments, leading to an accelerated degenerative change and eventual injury.

Studies have demonstrated that the most relaxed position for the hip is when flexed to 45°. Then the muscles at the back and front of the hip are balanced and the spine is able to retain its normal lumbar curve. Most people choose this position for sleeping – lying on their side with hips flexed to 45°.

Another example of this comfortable hip position is the posture adopted for horse riding. You can note how upright the spine is with the hips flexed to 50 to 60° and the body in perfect balance able to adjust its position as

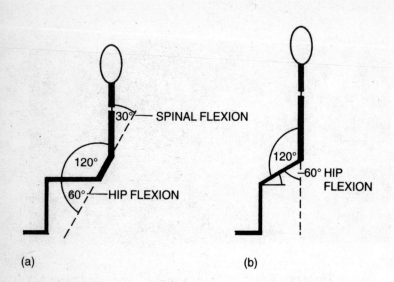

Fig. 5.6 Schematic comparison between (a) the traditional sitting position – note the 30 degrees of spinal flexion; and (b) the balanced sitting posture – note the erect spine. (Adapted from Mandal 1985).

required with the movement of the horse.

The best sitting position for balance of the pelvis and lumbar spine would show the hips flexed at 60° and the angle between the thighs and trunk at 120°. We can demonstrate this schematically (*fig.* 5.6). This represents a major departure from the traditional sitting posture based around the 90° angle.

There are recent styles of seating that have begun to incorporate this sitting posture, such as the kneeler chair and more traditional chairs with a forward tilt. These chairs have not found universal favour with designers and ergonomists. But try asking someone with back pain what

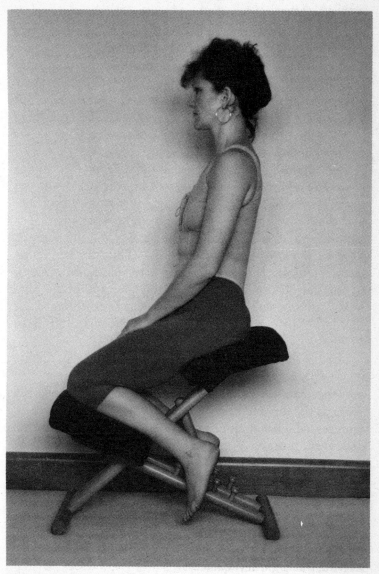

Fig. 5.7 Sitting on a kneeler chair.

they think! The forward-tilt chairs are far more comfortable for the spine and enable some people to continue work when they would not otherwise be able to do so.

The kneeler chair is not without some disadvantages and these are detailed in the next chapter. It will be a posture of choice for many people, and I believe that every office should have one available for use by its staff. This may help in assisting recovery from an injury, or for certain tasks, or just for postural variation.

The standard office chair with a forward-tilt mechanism has many postural advantages, without the disadvantages associated with kneeling. The angle of tilt is by necessity less than that of a kneeler chair, otherwise there is a tendency to slide forward on the seat or for the sitter to slide forward within their clothing. This can feel quite uncomfortable. The degree of slip is related to the amount of friction on the seat covering and the type of clothing worn. As a general rule, a seat with a fixed forward tilt should not be more than 10°, a variable forward tilt up to 15° and a kneeler chair up to 30°.

The degree of forward tilt does not necessarily dictate the sitting angle of the trunk to the thighs. This is also influenced by the height of the chair. The increase in the angle at the hip and knee that a forward-tilt seat produces requires a higher than usual seat to take advantage of the improved posture. A forward-tilt seat that is too low negates the effect of the forward tilt.

As a general rule a forward-tilt chair will be higher than a conventional chair and it is important to adjust the desk height and work station position to allow for this. This does not necessarily apply to a kneeler chair where the forward tilt can be maintained at a conventional height by altering the angle at the knees.

If we are serious about reducing the level of back pain in

society, we must move towards forward-tilt seating in an effort to reduce the build up of stress on the lumbar spine. I hope in the future we will see more forward-tilt chairs and more conventional chairs with a forward-tilt mechanism. At the moment these are relatively expensive. I hope that as they become more popular the price will come down to a level where it will be practical to have them in schools, universities and other institutions.

I am convinced that a little extra expense to ensure good-quality seating, appropriate to the individual, will pay dividends in better productivity, less time off, less pain and disability and happier people.

For the seating positions that enable a person to lean backwards, such as the cinema or theatre, or an interview situation, there is substantial research that a back rest can significantly reduce the stress to the spine. It produces a decrease in the disc pressure and reduces the amount of muscle activity required to maintain the posture. Leaning back against the back rest is an excellent posture for those people able to use it. These tend to be relaxing postures, or work postures where the visual attention is at or near eye level. Many chairs are designed with these postures in mind, such as the easy chair for watching television, the executive chair and the driving posture. These chairs often have a backward tilt of 5° to tip the occupant toward the back rest and prevent them sliding forward. This posture is discussed in the next chapter. However, a back rest is only of value if it is used, and a forward-leaning posture such as working at a horizontal desk makes little use of the back rest. A forward-leaning posture with a backward tilting seat is not only inadvisable, it is positively dangerous. The increase in disc pressure and the difficulty in relieving it is a recipe for back injury. The osteopathic clinics around the country are full of executives who are required to lean

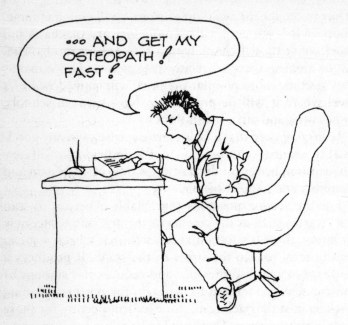

forward out of their comfortable chairs when they work at their desks and computers.

Being able to lean back against a back rest and stretch the spine and relieve the pressure on the discs is a very welcome postural variation for almost every sitting position, even if only for short periods.

JOINT COMFORT ZONE – SPINE, PELVIS AND HIPS
The angle between the thighs and trunk should be between 110 and 130° (see figure 5.6 on page 80).

The upper spine

The positioning of our head and neck is determined by the need to see what we are doing. The most balanced position for the head and neck is the erect position with a straight neck, looking straight ahead. This uses approximately 2 per cent of the maximum muscular strength of the neck muscles. A slightly forward-bent position of the neck requires about 10 per cent of neck muscle strength; a further flexed position about 17 per cent of strength. It is generally regarded that a continuous work situation should not use more than 4 per cent of muscular strength, otherwise it rapidly produces fatigue, and if continued, strain and injury. When we consider that in some occupational groups, such as medical secretaries, up to 50 per cent suffer from neck problems, it is clear that the arrangement of the work station to allow optimum positioning of the head and neck is vital.

The normal viewing angle is 10 to 15° below the horizontal and this is considered the resting position of the eyes with head and neck in a comfortable position. The eyes can comfortably accommodate vision 15° either side of the normal viewing angle. Any further change requires an altered posture of the head and neck which would eventually lead to postural stress.

It can be seen that wherever possible work should be inclined towards the vertical rather than horizontal. It should be above desk height and as close as practicable to the midline to avoid continual rotation of the neck. There is ample research to show that a copy holder, reading stand or inclined work surface can make a dramatic difference to the amount of postural discomfort. The work should be positioned at a comfortable viewing distance that does not strain the eyes or require an altered sitting position to see it properly. The focal length of the eyes is highly individual

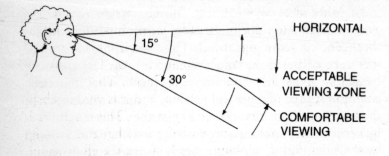

Fig. 5.9 The acceptable viewing zone.

and varies with age. It generally falls between 30 to 60cm, with shorter distances being usual in children and increasing with advancing age.

> OPTIMUM VISUAL ANGLE
> 10 to 20° below horizontal.

The shoulder

The positioning of the joints of the arm is crucial, with very little margin for error. Unlike the leg, the muscles that support the upper limbs are quite small with limited strength. They often have to work for sustained periods at a distance from the body. This creates considerable leverage and places these small muscles at a mechanical disadvantage requiring an increased workload and leading to a greater tendency toward strain.

The shoulders should hang loosely beside the body. There is a tendency during stressful work situations for the shoulders to tense up towards the ears. This puts an increased stress on the trapezius muscle – the large muscle band that joins the shoulder to the neck. This is a very common source of pain and tension, and it is vital to keep the trapezius muscle as relaxed as possible. This is achieved by keeping the shoulders low with the arms hanging loosely by the sides with a minimum gap between the elbows and the ribs. Any movement of the elbows away from the side of the body tends to stress the shoulder muscles on top of the shoulder blade that are required to maintain this position. Elevation of the shoulders or movement of the elbows away from the body is often caused by a work surface that is too high and can usually be remedied by raising the seat or lowering the work surface.

The upper arm should not tilt forward at the shoulder more than 10°. Any movement further forward increases the leverage and hence the strain. This is often done when the work is too far away from the body and requires over-reaching. It is a simple remedy to move the chair closer or move the work towards you.

JOINT COMFORT ZONE – SHOULDER

Arms hanging loosely by the side, forward from the body at an angle of up to 10°.

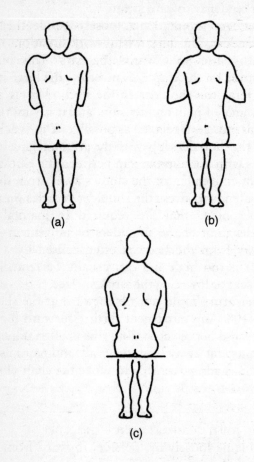

Fig. 5.10 Poor shoulder posture: (a) shoulders elevated;
(b) arms away from the body;
Good shoulder posture: (c) shoulders relaxed, arms by sides.

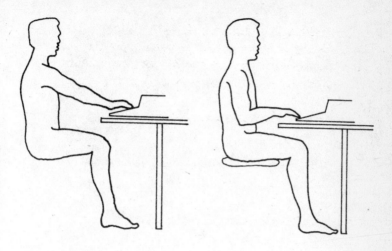

Fig. 5.11 (a) Poor shoulder posture – over-reaching.

(b) Good shoulder posture – arms close to the body.

The elbow and wrist

The elbow is most comfortably positioned at 90 to 100°. This is best achieved by positioning the work surface or keyboard at elbow height so that this position can be comfortably maintained. The wrist should be kept almost straight. A slight backward tilt is often required to allow positioning and manipulation of the fingers for tasks such as writing or typing. Sideways bending of the wrist should be minimised.

There is some evidence that the arm positions of the shoulder and elbow can be opened provided that the extended arms are well supported by a wrist or forearm support or are

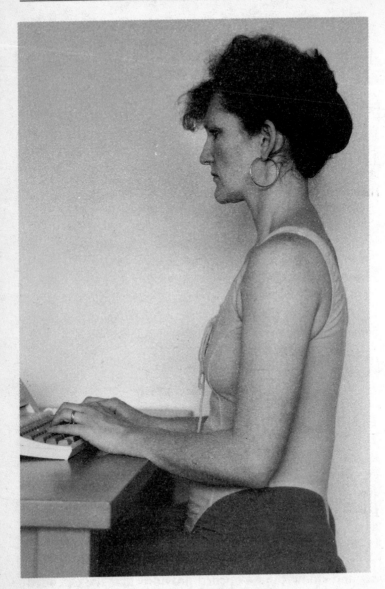

Fig. 5.12 Good shoulder, elbow and wrist posture.

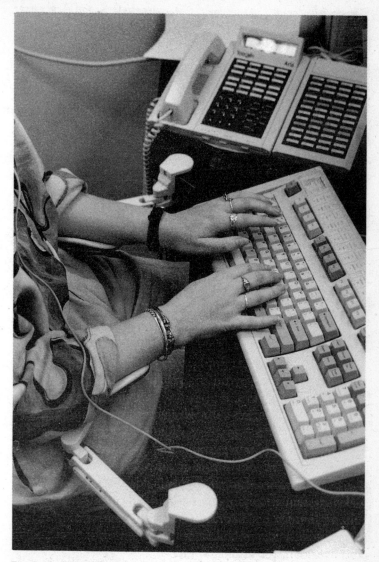

Fig. 5.13 A good forearm support can help reduce stress on the shoulders and arms.

resting on the work surface. Wrist and elbow supports should be adjustable in height and angle – and are only effective if they are used. If not used, they can become inconvenient and should be able to be removed or relocated.

JOINT COMFORT ZONES – ELBOW AND WRIST
Elbow – 90 to 100°.
Wrist – horizontal or backward tilt up to 20°.

The instructions described above apply mainly to a work station, where the computer screen is separate and placed at eye level and the keyboard can be operated by touch-typing, allowing separate placement at a comfortable working position. For more manual writing operations the work surface is best arranged a little higher with a downward slope towards the user, so that a balance is obtained between the need to view and the need to write. The recommended angle is 10 to 40°, with the lower angles for writing and the steeper angles for reading. The increased angle of the elbow in the writing situation is somewhat compensated for by the support of the work surface.

The knees

As the knees do not have a significant weight through them in the sitting position, the precise angle is not overly crucial. If the knees are straightened it tends to stretch the hamstrings, providing a backward pull on the pelvis. This requires a slumping of the lumbar spine in order to maintain the upright sitting posture. This is bad posture and overloads the lumbar spine.

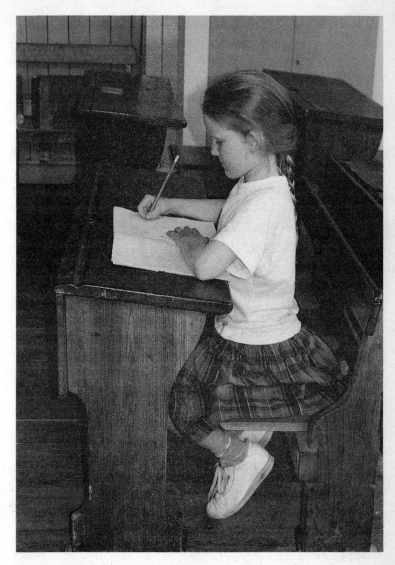

Fig. 5.14 A high sloping desk is the most suitable for reading and writing tasks.

> JOINT COMFORT ZONE – KNEES
> Knees – 60 to 120°.

The feet

In the sitting position the feet transmit a small amount of weight compared to standing, so the angle is not overtly crucial. It is desirable for the feet to be flat on the floor and the tendons to be in a relaxed position. If the feet are not able to be placed flat on the floor then a foot rest can be used to achieve this. A foot rest should be adjustable in position, and large enough to allow some movement of the feet and knees.

CROSSING THE LEGS

Crossing the legs while sitting is generally considered to be poor posture for the following reasons:

- It creates a pressure point on the buttocks.
- It creates a pressure point on the underside of the top leg which can restrict nerve and blood supply.
- It creates a pelvic twist.
- It creates a slouch in the lumbar spine.

In practice, sitting with the legs crossed tends to be quite uncomfortable and for that reason is usually self-limiting. There is evidence that as a postural variation it tends to increase the rate of fatigue rather than reduce it.

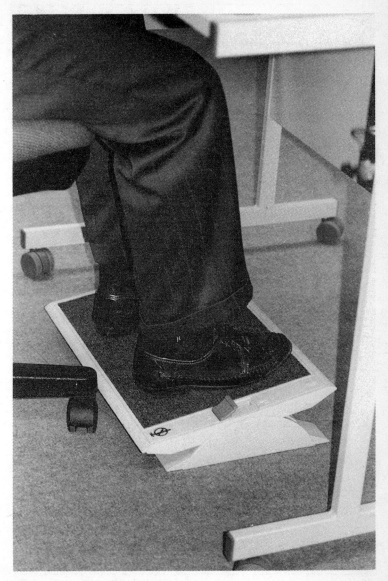

Fig. 5.15 A good example of a foot rest.

POSTURAL VARIATION

This chapter describes the ideal body position where there is minimal strain on the joints. I am now going to contradict that and say that there is no such thing as an ideal position! It is vital that sitting postures are dynamic and continually changing, that groups of muscle fibres do not have to work continuously but get periods of rest and recovery. It is important that the arrangement of a desk and chair allows for frequent postural variation and occasional stretching. If you are required to maintain a particular posture for a prolonged period of time without variation, as is commonplace with typing and computer work, the closer you can get to the joint comfort zones the less the strain will build up. In this situation regular pauses and breaks are *vital*.

This is a brief sketch of the principles of good sitting posture. The following chapters will show specific examples of good posture, what type of chair to use and how to arrange your desk and chair to best advantage.

JOINT COMFORT ZONES – SUMMARY	
Spine and pelvis	110 to 130°
Head and neck	erect
Visual angle	10 to 20° below horizontal
Shoulders	relaxed, by side, 0 to 10° in front
Elbows	90 to 100°
Wrists	horizontal or backward tilt up to 20°
Knees	60 to 120°
Feet	flat on the floor or foot rest

6

Good sitting posture – some examples

There is no such thing as the perfect sitting posture. We come in a variety of shapes and sizes, and what suits one person does not necessarily suit another. Different tasks require different positions. Even when a good position is found it requires frequent adjustments to maintain its degree of comfort.

There are, however, good and bad postures. This chapter will show three examples of good sitting posture. It will show why they are good and in what situations they are suitable.

When sitting for long periods, it is important that the sitting position can be varied throughout the day. This produces constantly variable stresses that allow the body's tissues periods of work interspaced with periods of rest. Ideally jobs should be planned to allow a variety of tasks throughout the day which would encourage regular changes of posture. As a result employees would become less fatigued, less bored, more content, more productive and have a reduced risk of injury.

It is vital that the seat and work station be planned to allow a variety of postures to be used.

DIFFERENT SITTING POSITIONS

A survey of office workers (Grandjean and Burandt, 1962) found that the employees used the following postures:

- 52 per cent sitting in the middle of the chair.
- 33 per cent sitting back in the chair.
- 15 per cent sitting forward in the chair.

Of the time spent sitting in these positions, 42 per cent of the time was spent leaning against the back rest and 40 per cent of the time with the arms on the table.

These figures show that office workers like to take a proportion of their weight off the spinal column as much as possible. They transfer weight and gain additional support by using the back rest or leaning on the table over 80 per cent of the time. This suggests that the traditional sitting posture, based on a series of right angles, is inherently uncomfortable for the spine.

I spend most of my working life treating people with spinal problems. I am well acquainted, personally and professionally, with the degree of pain, discomfort and disability that a spinal problem creates. It can make life very unpleasant. All the postures recommended in this chapter are based on the requirements for good spinal health.

THE UPRIGHT SITTING POSTURE

This posture is based on the work of Dr A.C. Mandal. It has been eloquently developed in his book *The Seated Man:*

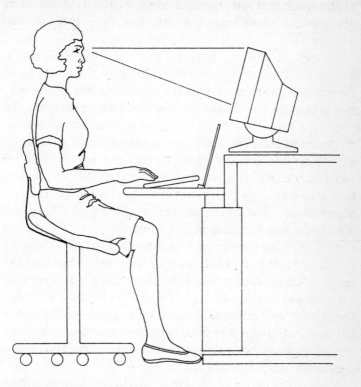

Fig. 6.1 The forward tilt chair provides a naturally balanced sitting posture.

Homo Sedens (Dafnia Publications, 1985).

To sit in the middle of a chair with an upright spine, leaning neither forward nor back, and maintaining the spine within its comfort zone (an angle between the thighs and trunk of 110 to 130°) requires a forward-tilted seat of 5 to 10°. Anything less than that will cause a compression of the spine and intervertebral discs which have not been designed to cope with this for sustained periods (see chapter 3).

This is the seating posture of choice for most work situations. It allows good configuration of the spine, from the lumbar spine up through the shoulders, head and neck. It is naturally well balanced and does not necessitate the continual use of methods to reduce spinal stress, such as slumping against the back rest or leaning forward on the work surface. It is an excellent sitting posture to allow postural variation. It has enough forward tilt to allow a forward-leaning posture for working at a horizontal surface such as a desk. If the chair is provided with a back rest it allows a backward-leaning posture.

The chair should be at a comfortable height allowing both feet to be flat on the floor (or foot rest). There should be no undue pressure under the thighs, nor a tendency to slip forward on the seat. It provides a comfortable angle for the knees and ankles, and it is a good position for circulation to the lower legs, with the extra muscle tone in the calves assisting to return venous circulation and reducing the tendency for varicose veins.

Ideally the chair should have a variable tilt mechanism to encourage postural variation within the forward tilt position. This can be spring loaded – where it is adjustable by shifting the body balance – or easily altered by a handle or wheel while in the sitting position. The optimum forward tilt is 5 to 10° but a good range is from horizontal to 15° forward.

In studies where subjects have been given the choice between a fixed forward-tilt chair and a variable-tilt chair, the subjects preferred the variable-tilt chair and made continual use of the variable-tilt mechanism. They tended to show an increasing number of movements and a greater

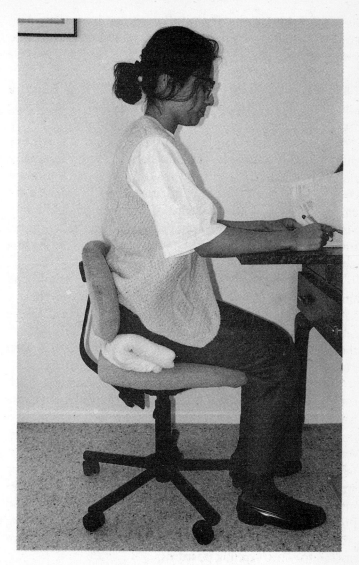

Fig. 6.2 A conventional chair can easily be modified to create a forward tilt seat.

degree of tilt as the time spent sitting increased. This suggests that a variable-tilt seat encourages increased frequency of postural change and a more comfortable range of postures. (Bendix, 1984 and 1985.)

This type of chair is suitable for a full range of work situations from a traditional horizontal desk, to a sloping work surface, to a typewriter or computer station.

While this is my working posture of choice, it is not one that is readily available. It tends to be the more expensive ranges of chairs that allow forward tilt as an option. A conventional chair can easily be converted to a forward-tilt chair by using a foam wedge. Some companies manufacture these and they are relatively inexpensive. A folded towel or blanket placed at the rear of the seat can have a similar effect.

Allowing the increased angle between the trunk and thighs requires a slightly higher sitting posture than a conventional chair. The work surface will need to be adjusted to accommodate this. The recommended height of the forward-tilt chair is with the front edge (the lowest point of the seat) level with the top of the kneecaps.

This type of posture will benefit from having a back support. There is ample research demonstrating that the use of a back rest reduces the pressure in the intervertebral discs and, by providing support for the lumbar spine, reduces the workload of the spinal muscles. The back rest need not be a large one. It should support the lower lumbar spine and be adjustable in height and tilt. The ideal inclination is 100 to 110° relative to horizontal. It should provide some support in the upright posture looking straight ahead, but is unlikely to provide significant support in forward-leaning postures.

FORWARD-TILT SEAT – SUMMARY

Spinal posture	good
Neck/head position	good
Shoulder/arm position	good
Knee position	good
Feet/ankle position	good
Visual angle	good

The forward-tilt seat provides a comfortable, well-balanced position with minimal physical stress. It allows good postural variation. It is an excellent office work, writing or study posture.

THE RECLINING POSTURE

This is a posture that requires leaning against the back rest. It is an excellent relaxing posture – television, cinema, theatre, etc. – and is suitable in work situations which allow constant viewing at eye level – driving, computer operator, etc. – that allow you to rest the trunk against the back rest. It is a posture that has been developed by Professor Etienne Grandjean and his colleagues and is well documented in his book *Fitting the Task to the Man – a textbook of occupational ergonomics* (Taylor and Francis, 1988).

Grandjean and his colleagues evaluated 68 VDU operators provided with an adjustable seat and work station, recording the preferred postures and subjective evaluations. While this study applies to VDU and computer

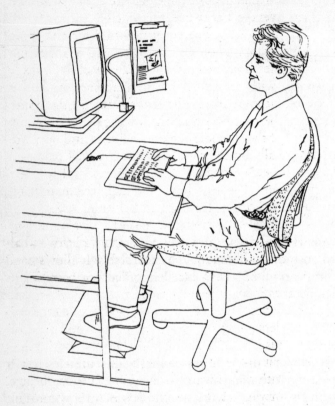

Fig. 6.3 The reclined sitting posture.

operators it also has relevance for other work situations, such as interviewing or telephone work, where the worker is not required to lean forward. It is very similar to the driving posture and airline seat posture (when reclined).

The subjects were provided with a chair with a nontiltable seat and a high, adjustable back rest. They chose to work at an average backward tilt of 104° (range 97 to 121°). This provided a degree of comfort for the spine reducing the compression of the discs and transferring weight onto the chair back. A high chair back is best for this posture, with an adjustable lumbar support and a convex thoracic support. In the work situation the upper back rest can be narrower than the lower portion to allow full mobility of the shoulderblades. The head and neck are situated vertically on the shoulders and are well balanced with a good viewing angle (9° below horizontal was the chosen position.) The legs have minimal weight bearing and can choose the most comfortable position.

This is an excellent relaxing position for the trunk and spine. It is well supported, allowing the muscles to be relaxed, with very little stress through the lumbar spine. For complete relaxation purposes the seat can be reclined further, such as in an easy chair when watching television. As the seat reclines there can be a tendency to slide forward on the seat, depending on the shape of seat and type of upholstery. This is usually compensated for by providing a 5° backward tilt of the seat on this type of seating. If using this posture with a backward reclined seat it is important not to lean forward at the desk – this is a very stressful posture, causing the lumbar spine to become compressed.

The reclining posture is comfortable for the trunk, but it leans the body away from the work surface and requires some forward reaching at the shoulders and elbows. This places stress on the relatively small muscles at the shoulders and arms if continuously required to maintain this posture, and they rapidly fatigue. When using this as a work posture it is important to have regular pauses and breaks to allow the hard-working muscles to recover and prevent the onset of fatigue.

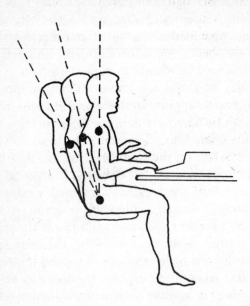

Fig. 6.4 The reclined sitting posture moves the body away from the work surface.

Stresses on the shoulder, elbow and wrist can be reduced by provision of an elbow or wrist support, or resting the forearms on the work surface. The forward reach of the upper arm requires a higher keyboard height than that usually recommended to keep the angle of the elbows within their comfort zones.

This can be a good posture for work at a well-designed work station. This is not a good posture for jobs that require leaning forward for tasks such as writing. The pressure in the lumbar spine and the spinal muscles soon builds up to undesirable levels, while the neck has to lean forward excessively to view the task, resulting in increased levels of neck tension. A seat with a forward-tilt option allows a simple adjustment into the upright posture previously described, if the task requires it.

The reclining posture – Summary	
Spinal posture	good
Neck/head position	good
Shoulder/arm position	requires careful attention
Knee position	good
Feet/ankle position	good
Visual angle	good

The reclining posture is an excellent posture for relaxing the trunk. It is suitable for tasks requiring viewing at eye level. It requires a well-designed work station and good work management.

Relaxing in the reclined posture

The reclining seat provides the best method of relaxing when sitting. The postural muscles are able to relax, the body is well supported, and it becomes a very easy thing to relax and even enjoy a post-prandial snooze!

An easy chair for relaxing usually provides a greater degree of backward tilt, with head and neck support. The chair back is larger to support the shoulders and arms. The upholstery is usually well padded with the emphasis on comfort rather than support.

These types of chairs are not usually good work chairs, they are not well designed for support in the work situation.

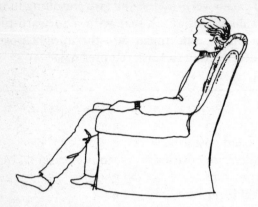

Fig. 6.5 Relaxing in the reclining position.

THE KNEELER CHAIR

As research has begun to show that the conventional sitting posture increases the pressure in the lumbar spine and can create serious back problems, people have begun to look at alternative chair designs. As outlined in the previous chapters, increasing the angle between the trunk and thighs when sitting reduces the compression of the lumbar spine and lowers the disc pressures. This discovery has provided the impetus for the development of forward-tilt seating. I am an enthusiastic advocate of the benefits of this type of seating and believe its widespread application could significantly reduce the ever-increasing incidence of low-back problems. When increasing the angle on a forward-tilt seat, there becomes a critical point when the sitter starts to slide forward on the chair, and the legs can feel quite uncomfortable having to resist this forward sliding force for long periods of time. This is where the kneeler chair comes into

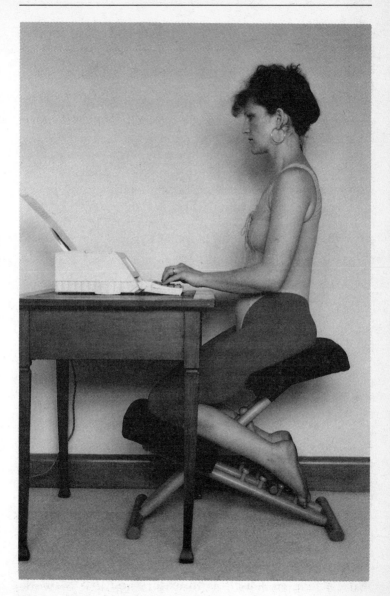

Fig. 6.6 Working with the kneeler chair.

its own. It provides a forward-tilt seat and a pad for the knees that prevent forward slide. There are a number of kneeler chairs available, but probably the best known is the Balans chair.

The kneeler chair allows an increased forward tilt of the chair and allows the hips, pelvis and lumbar spine to move into their optimum position, similar to that of riding a horse. It provides a balanced posture, reducing muscular stress and minimising disc pressure. It opens up the abdomen and chest allowing better breathing and better circulation. Better breathing brings about general relaxation and an improvement in concentration. It is the best available upright posture for spinal balance, and many of my patients suffering from back injuries, when provided with a kneeler chair, have been able to return to work earlier than would otherwise be possible when using a conventional chair. For people who suffer from chronic or recurrent back problems, this is the best sitting posture available to them.

A kneeler chair should have both sitting and kneeling pads adjustable for height. This allows adjustment at the seat height, the hip/spine angle and the distance between the seat and the knee pad depending on thigh length. The knee pad should be very well padded to prevent pressure on shin and knee bones. The chair should be on castors to improve mobility. The seat is usually tilted forwards anything between 10 to 30° and the kneeling pad tilted backward 10 to 20°.

As in the forward-tilt chair, this form of seating can provide a higher sitting posture and the desk or work station may have to be adjusted to suit this. To gain the most benefit from the improved spinal posture the kneeler chair is best used with a forward-tilting desk or work surface of 10 to 20°, allowing a better visual angle and an upright head and neck position. Unfortunately, it's not all good news and there are some disadvantages associated with the kneeler chair:

- Some people find the pressure on their knees and shins uncomfortable for long or continuous periods of sitting.
- The positions of knees and ankles are not very good and may restrict circulation to the lower leg.
- The feet are not well placed for use of foot pedals, such as on a sewing machine or dictaphone.
- They are a bit awkward to get on and off, and restrict mobility in an office environment.
- It is a relatively fixed posture with little opportunity for postural variation.
- They are socially unconventional.
- Some studies have shown that they can be fatiguing when used for long periods.

KNEELER CHAIR – SUMMARY	
Spinal posture	excellent
Neck/head position	good
Shoulder position	good
Knee position	poor
Feet/ankle position	poor
Visual angle	good

The kneeler chair will never replace the conventional chair, but it provides a very valuable alternative method of seating that comes into its own for people rehabilitating from a back injury. Some people find them ideal for short periods of sitting or tasks where an upright posture is required.

Are you sitting comfortably?

DRIVING

There is a significant relationship between driving and back injury. Men who spend at least half the time driving are three times more likely to develop an acute prolapsed disc. Truck drivers have an even higher risk, being five times more likely to have a prolapsed disc.

There is a direct relationship between the length of time spent in a car, the number of times getting in and out, and the risk of back injury. One study which interviewed regular drivers suffering from back pain asked them to list the factors which aggravated their symptoms. The results were:

- 93 per cent – sitting incorrectly.
- 50 per cent – reversing.
- 47 per cent – sitting in one position.
- 33 per cent – getting in and out.
- 20 per cent – operating the clutch.
- 10 per cent – inadequate lumbar support.

Vibration and road shock

The same general principles apply to motor vehicle seating as apply to other forms of seating with some additional factors that reflect its specialised nature. The most significant of these are the vibration and jarring from the road. This increases the rate of muscle fatigue and accelerates the compression of the intervertebral discs when compared with normal sitting.

There is a significant risk of injury after a period of driving when the discs are compressed, the muscles fatigued and the body is required to do lifting work, such as removing the shopping from the boot or unloading the van. The spine and its supporting tissues are in a very vulnerable state and easily strained. There are also additional demands made by the lateral forces involved in cornering. These require muscles to contract in order to maintain body balance and stability in ways which they are not designed for.

Driving posture

Driving is a very demanding posture. It involves simultaneous and precise movements of the arms and legs while maintaining constant visual attention.

The driver's posture is decided by the shape and position of the seat and the need to operate the controls. The hands are on the steering wheel from which they should not be removed unless changing gear. The feet are constantly required to operate the pedals. The driver has very little opportunity for postural variation due to the precise, continuous nature of the task.

The seat should be positioned so that the arms and legs are at a comfortable operating angle. The mechanism for adjusting the position of the seat should be easy to operate while sitting in the car. The seat height should be adjustable to provide optimum vision of the road and the instruments.

Pedal layout

The pedals should be in line with the hips. Operation of the clutch requires movement from the left hip and knee, and there should be a straight line from the hip to the knee to the action of the clutch. The brake pedal should similarly line up with the right hip and knee. When the legs are relaxed they like to splay out. The accelerator pedal should be offset to the right so the leg can remain relaxed while the pedal can be operated by foot pressure alone, with the heel resting on the floor. It is helpful to have a foot rest offset to the left to allow a relaxed position for the left leg when not in use and as an aid for postural stability. A car with pedals offset to one side can result in an uncomfortable sitting position and an awkward posture. This often occurs when the gearbox or wheel arch intrude into the driver's footwell.

Some drivers find that continual use of the clutch pedal can stress the spine and pelvis. If you suffer from spinal problems it may be worthwhile considering an automatic car.

It is important to position the seat so the legs are not required to overstretch for operation of the pedals. This would tend to backwardly tilt the pelvis and reduce the effectiveness of the lumbar support. The resting knee angle before operation of the pedals should be about 130°.

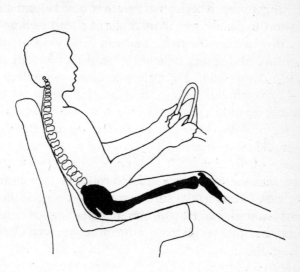

Fig. 7.1 Over-reaching for the pedals reduces the back support.

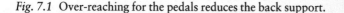

Holding the steering wheel

The steering wheel should be height adjustable and is best used in the lower range of its height, provided you can see the instruments clearly. The classic 'ten to two' position of the hands on the wheel, with its high arm position, involves a lot of neck and shoulder strain when driving for long periods. The upper arms should be able to hang beside the body, with an angle of not more than 20° in front, and the steering wheel should be held with two hands on its lower half (twenty to four).

Power steering is a definite asset and reduces con-siderably the awkward shoulder and trunk movements associated with parking in a confined space. Some cars have the steering wheel offset, so that it is mounted at an angle to the dashboard. This requires over-reaching with one arm – usually the right, and can produce a torsion in the thorax and spine, which can lead to postural stress. This is a design fault, that is less common in modern cars, but it is worthwhile trying to avoid this awkward sitting posture.

Head room

Ensure that there is sufficient head room, with a clearance of at least 10cm. Make sure that there is a good field of vision, unhindered by sun visors, shading or stickers. Ensure that the windscreen wipers adequately clear the

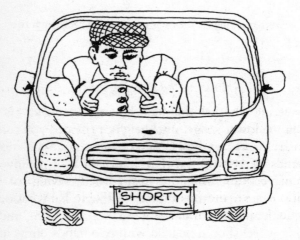

Fig. 7.2 Choose a car that suits your body shape.

section of the windscreen required for vision. For many years Volkswagen Golfs had windscreen wipers designed for left-hand drive in their right-hand drive cars and the wipers didn't clear the section of the windscreen that I needed to see out of. This produced significant visual and postural stress when driving in wet conditions.

If you are large or tall or have a long body, choose a car that suits your body shape. Too many people cram themselves into a small car and have to slouch with bad posture to drive effectively. One of my patients arrived driving a Honda Civic, which is normally a very good small car. He was six feet 10 inches tall and his head and shoulders had to compete with his knees to reach the steering wheel! It was a dreadful posture.

The seat

It should be firm as opposed to soft and very well contoured to suit your natural body shape. Cloth is the best material as it provides a degree of friction which helps maintain posture. Leather and vinyl are too slippery and less heat/sweat absorbent. The reclining position is the best for driving. This takes a significant weight off the spinal column and reduces the effect of shock and vibration on the muscles and joints. The back rest should be adjustable in angle, with an ideal driving position being 20 to 25° back from vertical. This should allow a comfortable reclined posture while still providing good arm and leg position, with the head and neck able to remain erect without having to 'crane' forward.

Lumbar support

It is very important to have an adjustable lumbar support to keep as much of the natural lumbar lordosis as is comfortable. An adjustable thoracic support is beneficial to provide support for the mid-back kyphosis. The more of the seat in contact with the spine in its natural curves, the greater the comfort and stability of the spine. It is very important to ensure that the lumbar spine is not in a slouched position, and this depends on good lumbar and pelvic support and not over-reaching for the foot pedals or steering wheel.

The seat should be adjustable to your size and shape, not vice versa. We are all different shapes and sizes, and it is important that seats are multi-adjustable to allow for this. It is important that the driver's seat be inclined slightly backwards. There is a tendency for the driver to slip forwards and the inclined seat helps to prevent this. It also facilitates the spinal support of the seat back.

It is generally better for a car to have an adjustable lumbar support rather than using an appliance. These tend to change the relationship of the sitter to the seat and head rest, reducing the support in other areas. In the absence of good built-in lumbar support, an appliance can be very helpful in maintaining a lumbar curve. It should be flexible so it can mould to the contours of the back and the seat. Air or liquid filled lumbar supports are not firm enough to provide adequate lateral stability when cornering. A rolled up towel can be used to good effect. It should be positioned at the belt line.

Lateral support

Both the seat and the seat back should have firm lateral support, i.e. support for the sides of the body especially when the car goes around corners. Ideally these would be adjustable to suit the shape of the driver. A tall driver requires more pronounced trunk support, while shorter drivers require better lateral support at the seat.

Head rest

A head rest is vital to support the head and neck and prevent whiplash in case of an accident. This can be lifesaving. It is not designed to support the weight of the head in the normal driving posture. It should be adjustable for height and its forward–backward tilt. In the normal driving posture it should be lightly touching the top of the neck and the back of the head without restricting mobility.

Rest periods

Driving is a very demanding posture with very little opportunity for postural variation. For this reason it is important to have regular breaks. I recommend 10 minutes for every one hour of driving. This should be used for some walking and some basic spinal stretches (see chapter 9).

Summary

When choosing a car people tend to be impressed by styling and performance. More attention should be given to a car that provides a good driving position with an adjustable seat designed to suit the driver.

ADJUSTABILITY OF THE DRIVER'S SEAT

Adjustment	Purpose
Forwards/backwards	for good arm and leg positions.
Height adjustment	for best visual requirements.
Seat inclination	for thigh support, and to prevent sliding forward.
Back rest inclination	to support the spine and help stability.
Lumbo-pelvic support	to keep a good lumbar curve and pelvic stability.
Thoracic support	to support the mid-spine.
Head rest	vertical and horizontal adjustment to support the head and neck in case of accident.
Lateral support	to provide stability to the body when cornering.

THE STUDENT

Modern school furniture is usually based upon:

- A low chair with a back rest and a flat or reverse-inclined hard seat.
- A low flat desk.

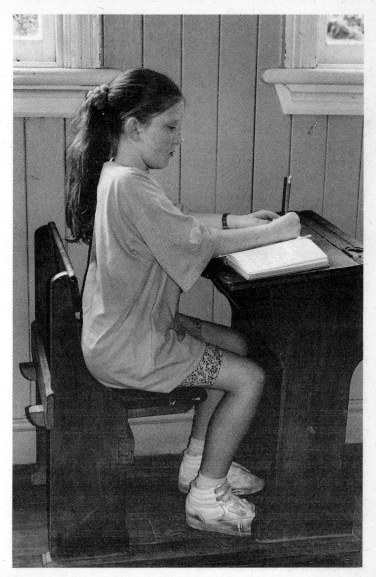

Fig. 7.3a The old-fashioned school desk.

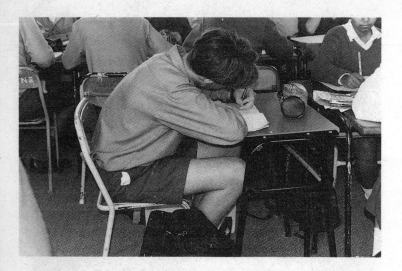

Fig. 7.3b The modern school desk.

School furniture design is often based on practical considerations such as the ease of moving and stacking, and the convenience of joining together.

The old-fashioned school desk with its high, inclined surface has largely been replaced by the low flat desk. Despite the evidence that children are substantially taller and exhibit growth spurts at a younger age than previous generations, school furniture seems to have shrunk.

The modern school chair provides a reasonable posture for listening to the teacher, looking at the blackboard and talking to friends when the child is able to lean against the back rest. It provides a dreadful posture when the student is required to read and write.

Children have to lean over the desk top to achieve a good

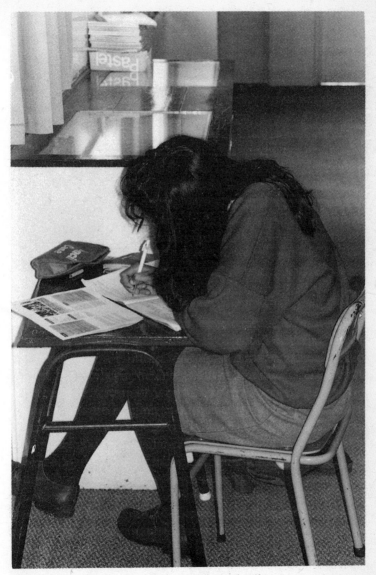

Fig. 7.4 The modern school desk encourages slouching.

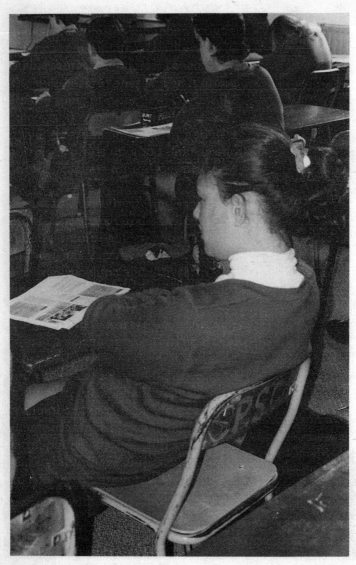

Fig. 7.5a Avoidance posture: slumping against the seat.

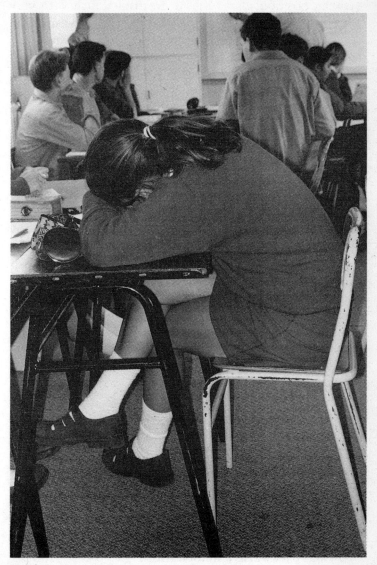

Fig. 7.5b Avoidance posture: leaning on the table.

viewing position. It requires a dreadful slouch with very poor posture. Fatigue rapidly sets in and concentration deteriorates. Close observation of children's posture has shown that they have developed a number of methods of reducing the postural stress. These include slumping against the back rest and leaning their elbows on the table.

Avoidance postures

These are not very satisfactory postures and tend to be quite uncomfortable, leading to the development of pressure points. The pressure points occur on the upper spine where it slumps against the back rest; the base of the buttocks where they catch the chair edge; and the bony elbows leaning on the table. These avoidance postures tend not to be held very long as they soon become uncomfortable. As a result students are often seen to fidget as they try to avoid discomfort and find a satisfactory position. These slumping and slouching positions are often regarded as poor posture, but are in fact a continual effort to find a comfortable position. This is nicely illustrated by *Fidgety Philip*:

Let me see if Philip can
Be a little gentleman;
Let me see, if he is able
To sit still for once at table.
But fidgety Phil,
He won't sit still;
He wriggles
And giggles,
And then, I declare,
Swings backwards and forwards,
And tilts up his chair,

Just like any rocking horse –
'Philip! I am getting cross!'

Struwwelpeter, Heinrich Hoffman, 1848

Spinal problems in school children

There is evidence that children suffer a substantial amount of back pain. Various studies have shown an incidence of back and neck pain between 20 and 35 per cent. It tends to increase in frequency with age as the education system becomes more demanding and height increases. One study (Fisk et al., 1984) showed that 56 per cent of teenage males and 30 per cent of females suffered from x-ray evidence of the spinal degenerative condition known as Scheuermann's disease. This is thought to be caused by long periods of sitting when children undergo growth spurts and is associated with back problems in later life (see pages 41–6).

I recently surveyed a selection of college students. There were 205 students aged between 13 and 18 randomly selected and asked to complete a questionnaire relating to any spinal complaints they had experienced over the previous 12 months. The results showed that an astonishing 94 per cent complained of spinal problems. This figure was consistent for both males and females and through the different age groups (forms 3 to 7). The figures were distributed as follows:

- 57 per cent described lower back pain or ache.
- 32 per cent described mid-back pain or ache.
- 53 per cent described neck or shoulder pain or ache.
- 55 per cent described headaches.
- 197 per cent total.

The 197 per cent total means that on average each student had aches or pains under two of the categories.

These figures were very similar for both sexes, with the exception of headaches where 69 per cent of female students and 45 per cent of males complained of symptoms. It is very difficult to determine causes of pain in a group such as this. In an attempt to find out if there were any relevant factors involved I asked them if they were made better or worse by certain activities.

Activity	Worse %	Better %	Neither %
Walking	19	24	57
Sitting in a chair at school or at home doing homework	71	4	24
Relaxing e.g. watching TV in an easy chair	14	45	24
Sleeping	18	61	21

In summary: 94 per cent of students in this study suffered from spinal complaints, of which 71 per cent felt they were made worse by sitting for school work. Spinal complaints are a significant source of pain and disability, as well as preventing many students from developing their full potential.

Do future generations of our children have to suffer these problems? I do not think so. I believe that sound ergonomic principles applied to seating provided in our schools and homes could dramatically reduce the incidence of adolescent spinal problems. This is the challenge that lies ahead for educationalists, furniture designers and manufacturers, parents and students.

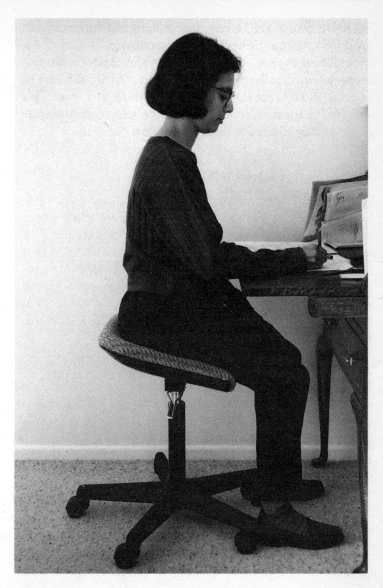

Fig. 7.6 A forward tilt seat gives a better spinal posture.

The remedies are simple: better designed furniture can produce a dramatic improvement in posture. We have little control over the type of furniture our young people have to use in schools, colleges and universities, but we are able to provide them with good-quality furniture at home. This will enable them to study more effectively, to concentrate better and help them to fulfil their potential.

Forward-tilt seats

The usual posture for reading and writing is a forward-leaning one. This enables us to view our work while seated at a desk or table. As outlined in the previous chapter, the best way to retain a healthy lumbar curve is to have a forward-tilt seat. This can be a fixed or variable forward-tilt seat or a kneeler chair. These are all excellent studying seats. The next best seating is a flat chair. On no account should a backward-tilting chair be used with a forward-leaning posture.

Chair back

A forward-leaning posture makes little use of a chair back. This tends to be used in the upright or backward-leaning postures. As a student studying in his or her own environment is free to get up for regular movement and postural variation, a chair back is not necessary to encourage this. A chair back is optional for a student's seat in the home environment. In the institutional environment where students are required to sit for defined periods of time, a chair back is useful for providing postural variation and the occasional stretch.

The desk

The seat determines the posture of the lower spine, but the position of work and the type of desk determine the posture of the head and neck. In order to maintain a good lumbar posture a backward-sloping desk should be used. A parent or teacher can instruct their children to sit up straight until they are blue in the face, but unless they provide them with adequately sloping desks children will always have poor posture and spinal problems.

For writing purposes the slope should be a relatively small one, approximately 10 to 15°. For reading the slope can be significantly increased – 45 to 60°.

For practical purposes it is sensible to have a desk that is suitable for both. This can be arranged so that there is a place for writing at the front of the desk, with a book rest towards the back of the desk.

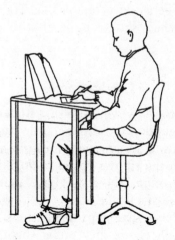

Fig. 7.7

A desk designed to serve as a dual-purpose reading and writing surface should have an intermediate slope of approximately 20°. A sloping desk should have a ledge at the base to prevent pencils, books and papers sliding off. There are adjustable boards that can be purchased which alter a flat desk to provide a sloping surface. These are also quite easy to improvise.

Height of chairs

The height of a flat chair seat should be approximately the level of the kneecaps (with shoes on). This allows a comfortable leg posture with feet flat on the floor and no pressure points under the thighs. Any lower than this will cause the knees to be higher than the hips, increasing the slouch in the lumbar spine and pelvis. Any higher than this would tend to lift the feet off the ground and create a pressure point where the thighs meet the edge of the chair. A foot rest can be used to counter this. The lowest edge of a forward-tilt chair should be level with the top of the kneecaps.

Height of desks

A desk that is too low will require a student to slouch in order to get a good visual distance from the work. When the person is sitting upright, with the arms hanging loosely at the side with the elbows flexed to 90°, the desk height should be approximately 5cm above the height of the elbow in the case of a flat desk.

There is evidence that as people become accustomed to using forward-tilt chairs they prefer slightly higher seats and desks. Children often prefer a higher relative desk height than that usually recommended.

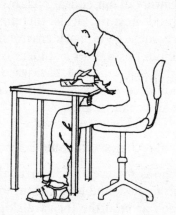

Fig. 7.8a A low flat desk encourages poor posture.

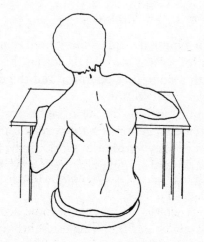

Fig. 7.8b A high flat desk can be awkward.

Summary

The existing furniture in our educational institutions is not designed for good posture. It is therefore even more important to provide a good work environment for home study. The optimum posture for a student is based around the forward-tilting seat and the backward-sloping desk. Ideally these should be positioned 5 to 10cm higher than traditional desk and chair heights.

THE SECRETARY

The secretary who is required to do manual clerical work is best served with a desk and table arrangement similar to the student, based around the forward-sloping chair and the backward-sloping desk. This optimises the posture of the lumbar spine and pelvis, and allows a good visual angle and position of the head and neck.

TYPING

The position for typing has quite specialised requirements. If using a word processor with VDU screen this has more in common with a computer operator and the details will be discussed under that section.

The best typing position is the upright posture. This, however, is often changed into a forward-leaning posture when looking at the keyboard or at work on the horizontal desk, or to a backward-leaning posture if a copy holder is provided to position the work at or near eye level.

The chair

The optimum seat is a height-adjustable, mobile office chair with a forward-tilt mechanism. This allows good upright posture. A good back rest which is height and tilt adjustable will assist with back support and allow ample opportunity for postural variation. The seat should be level with the kneecaps, and with the case of a forward-tilt seat the lowest point of the seat should be level with the top of the kneecaps.

The work surface

The table or desk surface should be level with the elbows when sitting with the arms hanging down and the elbows at 90°. The 5 to 10cm height difference of the typewriter keyboard will then bring the work surface up to the recommended level. If the work surface is planned for a good writing/reading height as previously recommended – 5cm above elbow height – the typewriter will raise the height to an uncomfortably high level which produces neck and shoulder stress. To compensate for this it is advisable to raise the seat to the extra height, and if necessary to use a foot rest.

There is ample evidence that using a copy holder can make a considerable difference to the degree of neck tension that develops. The copy holder should be set up to allow a good visual angle (just below a horizontal line from the eyes) and a good head and neck posture. It should be as close to the midline as is practicable.

The traditional typewriter with its requirement for feeding paper and returning the carriage used to provide opportunity for postural variation, but as the typewriter has become computerised and these functions have become automated, it is vital to ensure frequent postural changes and to have regular micropauses, pauses and breaks. Wrist or forearm support can be helpful in reducing postural stress.

Summary

Due to its continuous nature, typing requires a well-designed work station. This involves a height-adjustable secretarial-type chair with a flat or forward-tilt seat with good lumbar support. The work surface should be 5 to 10cm lower than that for normal writing. A well-placed copy holder should be used.

THE COMPUTER AND VDU OPERATOR

The advent of widespread computerisation in the early 1980s caused a new pain phenomenon. Many efficient secretaries who had not previously experienced difficulties with work became plagued by widespread and continuous pains in the hands, arms, shoulders, neck and spine. RSI became a household name.

It has become apparent that the design of the work station is a significant factor in the genesis of RSI. It is simply not good enough to plonk a computer on a desk and learn by trial and error. Someone spending a large portion of the working day at a computer deserves the best ergonomic arrangement of their work-space available. It requires good management and careful monitoring of their time, workload and work habits. If, by providing a good work station, workers can be more productive, more fulfilled, have better concentration and reduced fatigue and discomfort levels, the time and money spent on good ergonomic furniture will pay handsome dividends.

Choosing a posture

As outlined in the previous chapter, there are two suitable types of posture when working with computers.

The upright posture

This allows a balanced spinal posture with ease of mobility. It is ideal for mixed office work that requires movement and reaching, in addition to computer operations. It requires a flat or forward-tilt seat with a well-designed back rest.

The reclined posture

This is a more relaxed posture for the trunk, but requires a forward reach of the arms. It requires an office chair with a high back support and a backward-tilt seat. Its advantage is that it is the most relaxed position for the spine, but it allows little postural variation or mobility of the trunk. It requires a very well-equipped work station, which is properly adjusted to each user. It is not a particularly good posture for varied office work requiring frequent movement.

The chair

The best chair is one that allows both an upright posture and a reclined posture, with easy adjustment while seated. This chair would need to be height adjustable with a variable tilt seat ($-5°$ to $+10°$).It would require a high back rest, adjustable in height and angle, moving independently of the seat. Adjustable lumbar support would be an added advantage. This type of office chair with its advanced design and multi-adjustable features tends to be in the upper price brackets.

Most workplaces are likely to have an office chair with a low back rest. This is suited for the upright posture, which is a good position providing maximum mobility, good stability and minimum postural stress. The chair height should be adjusted so that the front of the seat is level with the kneecaps. With a forward-tilt seat the lowest point should be level with the top of the kneecaps. As a person becomes accustomed to a forward-tilt seat they often prefer a raised seat height. A backward-tilt seat used in the reclining position should have the highest part of the seat level with the lower kneecap. Never work in a forward-leaning position with a backward-tilt seat.

Back rest

The back rest should provide some support while sitting upright. There should be space below the lumbar support for the bottom to sit at the back of the seat, with the back rest providing maximum support just above the belt line. A well-adjusted back rest has significant postural advantages and reduces both the disc pressure and muscle tension in the lumbar spine.

The reclined position should have a high back rest adjusted so that it contacts as much of the back as possible and provides a good spinal support, while still allowing the operator to reach the work station comfortably with a good erect head and neck posture.

Arm rests

Arm rests can help with getting on and off a chair and can be used to support the weight of the arms when sitting. They should be height adjustable with some padding. They should support the elbow and forearm, but should not prevent the chair from being as close to the desk as desired. If they become a nuisance and are in the way, they should be able to be removed.

Wrist support

Most people like to use wrist or forearm support when they have the opportunity. This is not so much for use when actively keying but for support during pauses, such as waiting for computer responses or proof-reading work. To allow for this the keyboard should be adjustable in position on the work surface, with a space of at least 10cm from the edge of the work surface to the keyboard. It is often sufficient to use the work surface as a wrist/arm support. Alternatively supports can be purchased which fill the space before the keyboard and graduate the height up to the keyboard. See the illustrations on pages 90 and 91.

The keyboard

The keyboard should be between 640 to 780mm from the floor. The exact height is dependent on the combination of user and chair height. If it is to be used by a number of staff it should be adjustable in height between these parameters. The front of the keyboard should be no more than 20mm above the work surface and the height of the middle row of keys no more than 30mm. It should be inclined back toward the user 5 to 15°. This configuration allows good wrist posture while having convenient access to the work surface as a wrist/forearm support.

Copy holder

The use of a copy holder can make a marked difference to head and neck posture, and the muscle tension that can arise from poor posture. The ideal position for a copy holder is between the keyboard and the screen. If this is not possible it should be placed alongside the screen as close to

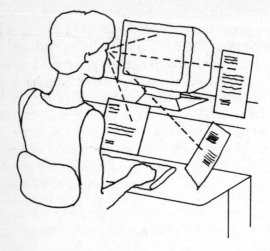

Fig. 7.9 Optional positions for the copy holder.

the midline as possible. In some situations where the screen is used infrequently the copy holder can be placed in the midline with the screen alongside.

Work surface

This should be height adjustable to allow the optimum keyboard position as previously described. If it is not adjustable, it is essential to have a height-adjustable chair and screen. There should be generous leg room, with sufficient depth to allow for alterations in leg posture. The work surface should be as thin as possible to ensure adequate height for the legs and maximum range of adjustability for the chair height. The recommended dimensions for knee room are 700mm wide by 550mm deep.

EXECUTIVE SEATING

The executive seat gives a modern example of the chair being used as a status symbol. It is large and sumptuous and has to reflect the user's importance. It is usually well designed for a reclining posture providing a high back rest with a good lumbar support. This allows the executive to lean back in comfort while dealing with personnel, or using the telephone, or pondering the current strategy. It is often not well designed for the upright or forward-leaning posture used for desk work or computer work. If these are an important part of the job, make sure that the chair is suitable for these tasks with a forward-tilt mechanism and a back rest that provides good lumbar support in the erect position. It can be difficult to find a chair that adequately combines both functions. It might be better to have a secretarial type chair available nearby when the situation requires it.

DINING

The position for dining is an upright forward-leaning posture, particularly if you enjoy pasta! The chair for this usually has a flat seat, ideally with some sort of padding to reduce pressure points. People generally sit at dining chairs for short periods, but when sitting for longer, they like to take the weight off the spine by leaning on the table with elbows or forearms or slumping against the back rest. The most important feature of a dining chair is that it has a recess underneath the back rest to allow the buttocks to sit

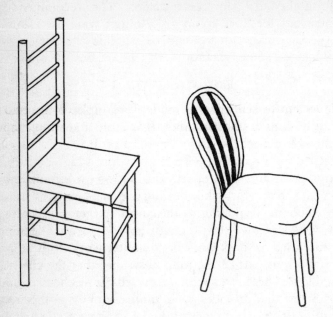

Fig. 7.10a A poor quality dining chair that doesn't allow for your natural curves.

Fig. 7.10b A better quality dining chair.

right back in the chair and still gain lumbar support from the back rest, which follows the spinal curves. The worst chair is a straight-back chair, which doesn't allow for the normal curves and forces the spine forward into a slouch.

A perfect meal can be spoilt by an uncomfortable chair, and many restaurants pay little attention to good seating. A comfortable chair which gives good support will invite you to linger over a meal, indulging in conversation as you enjoy the occasion.

RELAXING

A relaxing chair for reading or watching television, or indulging in some relaxation after a hard day's work, will allow you to recline back while your spine remains fully supported. It should have a high back, shaped for the lumbar lordosis and the thoracic kyphosis, up to shoulder level. It should slope backwards 20 to 30°. If the shape

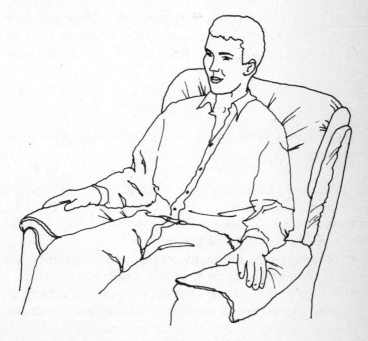

Fig. 7.11 The relaxing chair, built for comfort.

doesn't quite suit you, soft cushions can be strategically placed to allow better support. The seat should be flat or a slight reverse incline and should be well padded for comfort.

Arms are a very useful feature of a relaxing chair. They can aid in getting up and down, and can also provide very good arm support for some seated activities, such as knitting or breast feeding a baby. In these types of activities it is desirable to try and avoid stress on the shoulders and neck by having the arms unsupported. Try to transfer the weight onto the arm rest using cushions if necessary. My clinic becomes crowded with eager knitters at the onset of winter who, in the desire to finish their jerseys, spend too long with their arms suspended in front of them and their necks flexed to see their handiwork. When knitting or sewing take regular breaks, particularly if you are not used to it.

SOFAS

Sofas are often surprisingly uncomfortable. The most common faults are:

- Too low – difficult to get in and out of, forcing the spine into a round curve.
- Too deep – making it difficult to lean back for good spinal support. Cushions can help.
- Too old! – the springs have gone, and the lack of good support will force the spine into a slouch.
- Too low at the back – the back is not high enough to give support for the shoulders in the reclining position.

Look for a sofa with a seat that is just below the height at the kneecaps that allows you good low-back support while your feet are still on the ground, and with a back high enough to allow a comfortable reclining posture with your shoulders well supported. Never use a sofa or easy chair for a forward-leaning posture, such as doing paper work.

THE STOOL

This is one of the worst types of seating. Studies have shown this posture has greater disc pressure and spinal shrinkage than any other form of sitting. Stools usually have a hard edge that digs into the back of the thighs restricting circulation to the legs. When sitting on a stool, with its lack of back support, it is necessary to have an upright or forward-leaning posture, and this is best achieved by the forward-

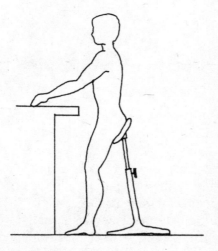

Fig. 7.12 An alternative to the stool – the sit-stand seat.

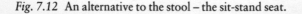

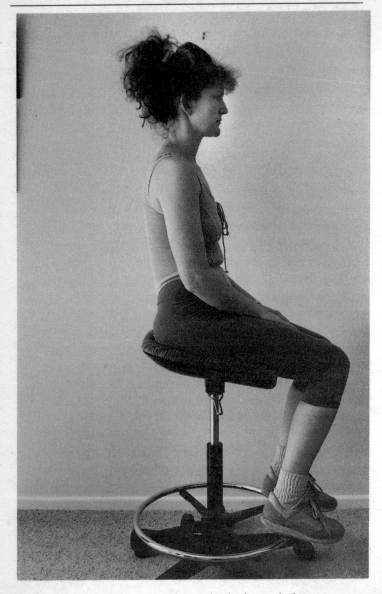

Fig. 7.13 Another alternative to the stool – the forward-tilt seat.

tilting seat which allows a higher than normal sitting position, is easy to get on and off and encourages excellent posture. A high forward-tilt seat is the preferred form of seating for people who require a higher than usual sitting position. A variation of this is the sit/stand seat or saddle chair, which is very useful for sitting at a work bench or tasks involving light manual work.

THE TOILET SEAT

Here I sit, alone and sixty,
Bald, and fat, and full of sin,
Cold the seat and loud the cistern,
As I read the Harpic tin.

Alan Bennett

The Anglo-Saxon empire seems to have considered the raised toilet seat and its comfortable sitting posture a part of decent civilisation. Notice the veritable library that many people have in the loo, which suggests a long sojourn on the 'throne'. Certainly, the character in this poem found it a comfortable place for contemplation. The modern toilet seat is built for comfort, rather than function.

The more traditional squatting position provides excellent physiological assistance for a bowel motion. The squatting position opens the pelvis and the sphincters. It also provides a marked increase in abdominal pressure. Both of these provide a powerful assistance to the natural process of defecation. This becomes all the more pertinent when we consider that our denatured, Westernised diet with its lack of fibre has rendered the whole process of the passing of our undigested products a more lengthy and difficult process than it was intended to be.

It is interesting to note that the same physiological advantages of squatting apply to the process of childbirth. It is heartening that the active birth movement and other avant-garde birth groups are recommending a return to this traditional birth posture.

8

Help!

This chapter will give advice for those people who may be suffering from pain and discomfort related to the postural demands of sitting, or the continuous and repetitive nature of the task that they are required to do.

As outlined in chapter four, the onset of discomfort usually progresses through various stages.

- Pain when working for long periods.
- Pain most of the time when working.
- Pain during and after work, and at some other occasions.
- Pain most of the time.

In most cases there is a progression from stages 1 to 4, and the warning signs become apparent early on. In some unfortunate cases, people seem unaware of stages 1 and 2 and become aware of the problem when it has already reached an advanced stage and becomes much more difficult to deal with.

Pain is your warning bell. The sign that your body is under stress. Never ignore it. Try and decide how best to deal with it to prevent it from becoming a serious problem. In the early stages all it may require is a break from the current task or a postural adjustment. In the more advanced stages it requires a concerted effort to find the optimum working postures, using good-quality ergonomic furniture, with careful management of work habits and workload.

PARTNERSHIP

The problem will not be solved by being stoic and battling away on your own. This will merely make the problem more chronic and more difficult to deal with at a later stage. Try and address the issues as soon as possible. At this stage it is best to involve other people as well as making a personal effort. The most effective approach is by involving three parties.

You

You are the one who has the most intimate knowledge of your problem, your pain levels, and the demands of the task that caused the problem. Experiment with solutions. Keep a diary recording when you feel better or worse and the possible reasons. Educate yourself as much as possible about the problem. Included in chapter 12 are questionnaires relating to the suitability of your work station and the overall picture of your work-related symptoms (see pages 270–6). This may help you to become clear in your own mind as to the extent of the problem and the solutions that may be required to assist you. Take photocopies of these questionnaires and give them to people who will be assisting you, such as your GP, therapist or employer.

Your employer

It is important to make your employer aware that you are suffering discomfort at an early stage. The employer has legal obligations to provide you with a work station that is suitable both for the task and the person using it. The Management of Health and Safety at Work Regulations are quite clear in this regard. They require employers to:

- Assess the risk to health and safety of their employees.
- Put into practice health and safety measures following the assessment.
- Set up emergency procedures and appoint appropriate people to assist with health and safety measures.
- Give employees staff training and information about their work station and its health and safety risks.

The Health and Safety (Display Screen Equipment) Regulations 1992 came into force in January 1993. These very thoroughly describe the minimum standards expected of employers. All work stations put into service on or after 1 January 1993 must meet the regulations as described. All work stations put into service on or before 31 December 1992 must meet the requirements not later than 31 December 1996.

The Regulations themselves are quite difficult reading. I have edited them to provide the key information in a more approachable form. These are included in the appendix, together with information on how to obtain a full copy of these or any other regulations published by the Health and Safety Executive (see pages 289–95). The enlightened employer will go to great lengths to ensure the well-being

of the staff and their ability to work effectively. They have
the opportunity to alter your work role, to include more
varied types of work and to avoid continued postural
stresses. They may already have a strategy for dealing with
work-related problems involving seeing the appropriate
medical personnel or enlisting the help of specialists such as
occupational health nurses or ergonomic specialists.

Try and keep your employer as informed as possible
about the problem and the steps you are taking or the
changes you feel are required to assist you. Try and do this
in a non-threatening way, giving them the opportunity to
assist you in overcoming the problem.

There are three very persuasive reasons why it is worthwhile for an employer to take the time, effort and expense
to ensure that an employee is working in a comfortable,
ergonomically suitable workspace:

- Staff morale – contented staff working in a comfortable
  environment have reduced absenteeism. They have
  reduced rates of sickness, stress-related problems and
  musculoskeletal pain. A well-motivated work force in a
  good environment will have a reduced staff turnover.
- Efficiency – provision of an ergonomically designed
  work space can dramatically increase office efficiency.
  In one study where a VDU work station designed
  according to commonly accepted ergonomic practice
  was compared with one that broke most of the guidelines, performance was 25 per cent higher in the
  ergonomically designed work space.

  In another study, the efficiency of data entry staff at
  Singapore airlines was compared before and after
  ergonomic changes, and relatively inexpensive changes
  produced a marked increase in productivity. The
  changes included an improvement in lighting, pro-

vision of copy holders and foot rests, and more frequent rest pauses. The performance (measured in keystrokes per hour) increased by 25 per cent and the error rate reduced from 1.5 per cent to 0.1 per cent. There was also a dramatic reduction in the incidence of musculoskeletal pain.

- Cost savings – these are a result of the improvements in staff morale and efficiency. By reducing absenteeism and staff turnover there are considerable cost savings to be made in sickness benefits, hiring replacements and staff training. The continuity of personnel produces an improvement in workplace efficiency. It simply becomes easier to produce a better-quality product and provide a better service.

Improvements in efficiency may reduce overall staff costs, and there is the possibility of taking advantage of new opportunities created by improved efficiencies and lower cost structures.

CHECKLIST FOR EMPLOYERS

- Do you have adjustable chairs, work surfaces, keyboards and screens?
- Are the temperature and humidity comfortable at all times?
- Is the lighting adequate, with minimal reflection or glare?
- Do you allow your employees to work at a comfortable pace in a relaxed atmosphere, without continual deadlines?
- Do you encourage job variation, with regular breaks when keying for long periods?

Included in chapter 12 is a work station assessment

questionnaire for you to fill in (see pages 270–2). This may help you become clear in your own mind as to the changes required to improve your working conditions. You may like to provide a copy of this to your employer or anyone given the responsibility of assessing your work station.

Dealing with a difficult employer

The larger employers are likely to have made some effort to address the health and safety issues of their work force and to implement the requirements of the Regulations. Many smaller employers have probably never considered it, and the first time the issue is addressed is when an employee starts to develop some symptoms.

In these cases the employer needs to become aware of the problems and the solutions required. The benefits as outlined here and the requirement of the Regulations should be persuasive enough to encourage most employers to take the issue seriously. There will always be occasional employers who are slow to accept the inevitable and who make little attempt to educate themselves regarding the scope of the problem and the reforms it requires. They may even try and 'blame' the employee as being the architect of their own misfortune in an effort to deflect responsibility. Remember that you are not the only person to suffer these symptoms and neither will you be the last. It may be difficult to deal with a reluctant employer, but by doing so you will be helping other employees now and in the future.

If you find your employer is inclined to blame you for your problems and to ignore the information you have provided, enlist support. In the first instance this could be your supervisor or other employees, or it could be a letter or phone call from your doctor, therapist or an occupational health nurse. If these still meet with no success, approach the relevant trade union to help make your employer aware of his or her legal obligations.

Try and be diplomatic in your dealings with your employer. Aim to enlist his or her support rather than feel you have to do battle with him or her. If you have difficulty in dealing with your employer directly, write a letter outlining your concerns. It is a good idea to keep a written record of all efforts you have made to approach your employer.

The very worst thing you can do is suffer in silence. You owe it to yourself, your future work prospects and future employees to make your employer aware of the problems you face and to try and assist him or her with finding the solutions.

Your doctor or therapist

Some kind of medical or therapeutic assistance can often be a key factor in overcoming these postural or overuse problems. Probably the best starting point is your own GP. Try and explain how long you have had the problem, how and when it started, when it causes pain, what makes it better or worse. Try and give him or her as much information as you can. Doctors have a broad knowledge of a wide range of medical conditions and can often provide a different perspective to the problem. They will ensure that there is no serious medical problem responsible for some or all of your symptoms, such as an inflammatory arthritis or an infection. They may arrange some further investigations such as x-rays or blood tests, or refer you to a specialist for an expert opinion.

A thorough physical examination is important. Although only one part of the body may be causing the pain, there are often other areas that are dysfunctional. For example pain in the forearms is a common symptom caused by overuse or an awkward posture at a keyboard, leading to muscle strain. The extra muscle tension may produce wrist and elbow stiffness. There would also probably be some involvement at the neck and shoulders as they attempt to compensate for the problem by increasing their workload. Though there may be a limited pain site initially, there are usually other regions that are under strain but not yet symptomatic. As the condition progresses these sites start to become increasingly involved and become painful. It is important that the GP or therapist takes a broad approach to the problem and ensures the entire body is functioning better, rather than just an isolated joint or muscle group.

Your doctor may be able to give you valuable advice concerning management of your condition, such as the advisability of time away from work, reducing working hours, exercises or further treatment.

If it has reached the stage where you have consulted your GP, usually some kind of further treatment is necessary. Your GP will have a referral network and will be able to refer you to someone who may be able to help you. Alternatively, you may decide to consult someone on your own initiative. Speak to other people in the office or to people who have had similar problems; they may be able to suggest a therapist who was helpful and has experience dealing with similar cases.

TREATMENT

There is no one treatment that suits everybody and it can be a personal exploration to find out which is the most appropriate therapy for you. This section will outline some of the treatments available and how they might help.

Ensure that the therapist is properly qualified for their

job (it's not always the case) and that they are registered with their professional organisation. This is to ensure your safety and that the therapist meets recognised standards of practice, ethics and competence.

Look for a practitioner who has a broad knowledge of muscles and joints and the way they work, with some experience in the type of problem you have. Ask them questions to make sure that they offer the kind of service you require. Try and ensure that they take a broad approach to the management of your problem, incorporating exercises, self-help techniques, postural advice, looking at the way your body works as a whole, rather than just isolating and healing a specific muscle or joint.

The practitioner should be able to make a clear diagnosis and give you some idea of how much treatment is required. All treatments used should be fully explained and any side effects made clear. Informed consent is an important part of medical ethics.

Treatment should have a logical sequence. If you are not showing some signs of improvement after four to six treatments, it is probably not going to help. Progress is usually graduated and don't expect to get better suddenly after a defined number of treatments.

Look for a practitioner who is able to give some idea of how to manage and prevent the problem in future, rather than require ongoing treatment to maintain the progress made. You may occasionally require some follow-up treatment after an extra workload, period of stress or some trauma, such as a car accident or a fall. Once you have suffered from these types of postural or overuse problems, you can become more sensitive to repeat occurrences, which should be addressed promptly.

CHECKLIST FOR YOUR THERAPIST

- Are they qualified and members of a professional organisation?
- Do they perform a thorough physical examination, looking at the whole body not just the localised area?
- Are they knowledgeable? Do they have an interest in the type of problem you have?
- Do they give self-help advice, with exercise, postural advice and advice on preventing recurrences?
- How much does it cost per visit? How often will they want to see you?

Anti-inflammatory drugs

These are the most commonly prescribed medication for muscle and joint injuries. They are highly effective in reducing pain and inflammation. The full name of this category of medicines is non-steroidal anti-inflammatory drugs (NSAIDs). The most common commercial names are: voltaren, surgam, dolobid, brufen, synflex, oruvail, indocid, naprosyn and feldene.

They are generally prescribed as a course of treatment and are most effective for chronic conditions when taken regularly. They can be taken symptomatically, i.e. taken as required during a painful episode or a sudden exacerbation of the symptoms. They should be used with caution. They are not a form of therapy, but they reduce the symptoms of pain and discomfort. Pain is a warning sign and by removing it it is very easy to continue a harmful activity and aggravate the problem, while under the mistaken belief that you are improving. Continued use of NSAIDs may have the effect of allowing you to turn what was a minor problem into a chronic problem that becomes difficult to treat by allowing you to continue to produce the strain that caused the injury in the first place. Make sure that you are addressing the cause of the pain and seeking the appropriate treatment by obtaining an adequate diagnosis and treatment plan in addition to using this medication.

Side effects

The most common side effects are those affecting the gastro-intestinal tract, including pain, nausea, vomiting, diarrhoea, cramps and excess acidity. These can progress to ulceration and bleeding. Less common side effects are skin rashes, kidney damage, blood disorders, headaches and vertigo. If you suspect any side effects, discontinue the medication and consult your GP.

Gels

Many anti-inflammatories are now available in the form of gels which are applied to the skin and absorbed into the local tissues. They produce a lower blood concentration of the active ingredients and have a much reduced incidence of side effects and toxicity. They can be very effective in reducing pain and inflammation, particularly where the tissues are easily accessible to the skin, such as wrist, forearm and neck. They should not be used habitually without ensuring a satisfactory diagnosis and that the cause of the condition has been addressed.

Side effects

Local irritation such as redness, rash and itching. Discontinue if these occur.

Corticosteroid injection

Some GPs and specialists favour the use of local injections of corticosteroid into the site of injury. This provides a powerful anti-inflammatory effect that can significantly alleviate pain and swelling. If the injection is well sited, the period of relief can last for four to six weeks. Once again, by suppressing pain, part of the body's alerting system for tissue trauma is removed and it becomes easier to continue an injury-promoting activity. Corticosteroid injections should only be used if there is an adequate diagnosis and the cause of the complaint has been fully addressed. It is generally recognised that corticosteroid injections should not be used repeatedly.

Side effects

Injections into tendons are not advised. These have been associated with tissue degeneration and increased risk of rupture. Injection into joint spaces has been associated with breakdown of the joint cartilage. Local side effects – thinning and discolouration of the skin.

Surgery

Surgery has a very small place in the treatment of RSI and postural-type problems. It should only be considered as a last resort, and even then it is advisable to proceed with caution. Surgery is most appropriate in times of trauma, when bones become fractured or dislocated. With gradual-onset problems such as RSI and postural problems, which involve mainly soft tissues, surgery is rarely indicated. Cutting through soft tissues causes scar tissue which can exacerbate any functional problems in that region.

Someone who has had RSI for a considerable period of

time often seems to develop increased sensitivity of the nervous system and can be a very poor responder to surgery – it can make them worse. Surgery may be of value where there is nerve pressure, such as in carpal tunnel syndrome in the wrist, or thoracic outlet syndrome, causing numbness or muscle weakness. Make sure that the nerve pressure is responsible for most of the symptoms, not just a small part of them, and as a general rule try non-invasive therapy first. If in doubt seek a second (or third or fourth!) opinion. If conservative treatment fails you have lost little; surgery causes permanent change.

Massage

This is a very effective form of treatment to help a tired, aching muscle. It is best performed along the length of the muscle fibres using some sort of lubrication such as baby oil or vegetable oil. It must be done deep enough to penetrate beneath the skin and underlying layer of fat.

When performed by someone skilled in its use, it can be very beneficial at all stages of overuse or postural injury. A few simple massage techniques can be learnt by a friend or partner, and providing they are not actually causing pain, they are likely to achieve some benefit in reducing pain and assisting relaxation. Some areas of the body are easily accessible for self-massage. Simple massage techniques for self-massage or massage by a friend will be described in the next chapter.

There are some specialised forms of massage that concentrate on particular pressure points such as acupressure, shiatsu, neuromuscular and rolfing.

Benefits of massage

- Improves the circulation to the muscle.
- Assists the removal of waste products from muscle spasm and inflammation.
- Assists in relaxation of the muscle (and the person!).

Mobilisation

Joints that are constantly used within a limited range of movement and are subject to muscle tension often become stiff and dysfunctional, producing strain. This is a common finding in RSI and postural problems. Mobilisation is the loosening up of these joints to try and improve their function and return the mobility to its normal levels. This can be achieved by doing exercises, such as yoga or stretches, but when performed by another person the technique is known as mobilisation. It is a very important component in the treatment of a joint problem and requires a specialised knowledge of joints and their soft tissues. It is best left to appropriately qualified practitioners.

Manipulation

This is a highly specialised form of mobilisation where a joint is taken slightly beyond its normal range of motion. This causes a change of pressure in the joint capsule and is usually accompanied by an audible pop or click. This seems to produce a number of effects:

- An improvement in mobility.
- A reduction in muscle spasm.
- A reduction in pain.

These effects seem to be produced by influencing the nerve fibres around the joint and stimulating the release of endorphins – a natural pain modifying substance produced by the body. Manipulation is a valuable tool in the treatment of joint problems and is particularly helpful for spinal complaints. It requires a high degree of skill to perform it safely and effectively and should be left to the experts. Osteopaths and chiropractors learn manipulative techniques at undergraduate level and as a general rule are well educated in their effective use. Physiotherapists and GPs now have the opportunity to attend post-graduate courses in manipulative techniques and often become effective manipulative therapists.

Osteopathy

Osteopathy was founded in Kirksville, Missouri, USA in 1874 by Dr Andrew Taylor Still. It is a system of therapy that lays its main emphasis on the structural and mechanical problems of the body. Osteopaths believe that structure affects function. They consider that the body works as a functional unit, so they look at the whole body in addition to the injured part. An osteopathic consultation involves a detailed case history and a physical examination involving palpation and testing of joints and soft tissues.

Osteopaths use manual therapy as their principal form of treatment. This usually involves some soft tissue release techniques, some mobilisation and some manipulation. An osteopath will usually give advice on self-help techniques, such as exercises, posture, hydrotherapy or ice packs.

Osteopaths were for a long time regarded as 'alternative' therapists and as such many GPs were reluctant to work with them. This is no longer the case – osteopaths are now recognised as practising a valid and soundly based form of therapy, and most GPs and specialists are happy to work with them. Most of an osteopath's workload tends to be dealing with spinal problems, but the approach works equally well with other joint and muscle problems.

Chiropractic

Chiropractic originated in mid-western USA back in 1895 when it was developed by Daniel Palmer. It has a philosophy very similar to osteopathy and in many respects the two professions are very similar, both being based on the belief that the structure of the body is intimately related to its function and both using manual techniques to restore and balance the musculoskeletal system of the body. Both therapies involve four or five years' full-time study, and most colleges now offer degree courses.

There are some differences between the two professions that are still apparent. Chiropractors emphasise the use of x-rays for diagnosis, and as a general rule focus on the use of spinal manipulation. These are generalisations. Treatment can often vary quite considerably from one osteopath to another, or one chiropractor to another. Practitioners tend to use the techniques that they feel comfortable with, based on their education, experience and the type of patient they treat.

A practitioner should always be willing to answer questions about their approach to a particular problem or the type of techniques they use.

Physiotherapy

Physiotherapy covers a wide range of treatments. The graduate physiotherapist will have received training in a broad area of therapy, ranging from stroke rehabilitation, post-surgery rehabilitation, pulmonary (lung) problems, as well as the overuse and postural problems that are the subject of this book. A physiotherapist will often use electrical equipment, such as ultrasound, interferential, microwave, magnetic therapy, etc. These are designed to enhance the natural healing mechanisms of the body. A physiotherapist specialising in musculoskeletal problems will often have done post-graduate study incorporating manual techniques such as mobilisation and manipulation.

Exercises are often an important part of physiotherapy treatment.

Acupuncture

This can be a very valuable form of treatment for muscle and joint pain. It is no longer regarded as an esoteric form of Eastern medicine that works independently of our Western knowledge of science.

There are a number of therapeutic avenues by which it seems to work.

- A needle placed in a tissue increases the circulation to that area for up to one week.
- It can directly relax a tense muscle by influencing special sensory fibres in the muscle.
- It can reduce pain by influencing the state of excitability of nerve fibres.
- It promotes the release of endorphins, the natural pain modifying substances produced by the body.

If you attend an acupuncturist make sure they are well qualified and have good standards of hygiene. An acupuncturist with a good knowledge of muscles and joints and their common trigger points will produce better results than one whose knowledge is limited in this area.

Acupuncturists talk about the rule of thirds: one third of people respond very well; one third respond quite well; one third are poor responders.

I have found acupuncture works best when combined with muscle release, mobilisation and manipulation.

The Alexander Technique

This is a system of postural awareness that aims to make people more conscious of how they use their bodies. Alexander teachers follow the maxim: use affects functioning. An Alexander teacher will take a student through a series of movements and postures, making them aware of the need for good posture and muscle balance. It can be very beneficial for postural problems related to the prolonged sitting position.

EXERCISES

Exercise plays a very important part in the treatment and rehabilitation of overuse and postural injuries. Your GP or therapist should be able to advise you on types of exercise that may help you recover from these problems, reduce the likelihood of recurrence, and better still, prevent them in the first place. Exercise neatly divides into two sub groups:

- Exercise to improve mobility.
- Exercise to improve strength and fitness.

Both these types of exercise are beneficial, and the particular types of exercise and the balance of these two categories varies with each person and their relative fitness.

Someone who is naturally hypermobile or loose jointed generally has poor muscle tone and joint instability and can be prone to joint strain. They tend to benefit from exercise that improves the muscle tone and stabilises the joints. This tends to be repetitive exercise within a defined position of joint motion – where the joints are not overstretched. Good examples of this type of exercise are: jogging, swimming and gym circuit training.

A person who has a tendency to be naturally stiff and struggles to touch their toes will generally have better muscle tone and a tendency towards tight joints that are restricted in their range of motion. A stiff joint generally works less efficiently and is more likely to build up stress and strain. This person will benefit from exercises that are going to increase the range of joint motion while building up fitness. Examples of these types of exercise are: yoga, stretches and gymnastics.

Advice on specific exercises for joint problems is covered in the following chapter. The health-promoting benefits of exercise and advice about starting an exercise programme are covered in chapter 10.

RELAXATION

There seems to be a relationship between mental stress and physical stress. People who work in a stressful environment or have a difficult personal life seem more prone to developing muscle and joint problems and often find it more difficult to recover from them once they have developed a problem. The more tense a muscle is when in its resting state, the less workload is required to make the muscle feel fatigued and achy.

Pain can be very stressful and people who have pain much of the time find it very difficult to relax. They become very tense and can often be labelled as neurotic or even depressed. During the 1980s, when it became apparent that RSI was a widespread phenomenon and many objective scientists were unable to find an easily recognisable marker to make a diagnosis (such as a positive blood test or an abnormal x-ray), it was very common to label these problems as psychogenic (originating in the mind). In most cases this was erroneous, and it continues to be a cause of mis-diagnosis with people in chronic pain. It is entirely understandable that people with persistent pain, who become frustrated by the inability of the medical establishment to fully understand and treat their problem, tend to become a bit distressed. In most cases this is part of the symptoms, not the cause of the problem.

Reducing muscle tension

When a joint becomes painful there is usually a protective reflex that tightens the muscle around the joint to try and splint it and prevent it from undergoing further trauma. A part of this is involuntary and in an acute injury is not under conscious control. In a longstanding injury this can be more a matter of habit, and the persistently tense muscles become fatigued, develop trigger points and start to become a source of pain themselves.

It is important to be able to relax the tissues involved in a painful joint so as not to accelerate the fatigue process. This can be done by an isometric contraction. An isometric contraction is when you tense the muscle without changing the position of the joint involved. An isometric contraction of the forearm involves clenching the fist. A good relaxation technique for the neck and shoulders involves shrugging the shoulders up towards the ears, holding them for a few seconds and then releasing them as quickly as possible.

This is an excellent relaxation technique when working at a desk or computer, where the shoulders and neck often become tense without people realising.

I generally suggest that the isometric contraction is held for three seconds and then released as quickly as possible, while at the same time breathing out and consciously relaxing the part of the body, feeling it become looser and heavier. This can be repeated three to four times with a five to ten second pause between each one to allow for the relaxation. The tissues gradually become more relaxed each time. With a little practice it soon becomes very easy to consciously relax the affected joint. There is an additional benefit to this exercise as isometric contractions are a good way of improving the circulation and muscle tone around a joint.

This is an excellent principle of relaxation when there is a local problem confined to one part of the body.

Relaxation techniques

When people are generally overstressed or tense, or have developed tension as part of a chronic pain pattern, they benefit from relaxation techniques that promote their inner state of calm and reduce their levels of anxiety. There are many ways of doing this and it can be helpful to find one that works for you.

Heat can be very relaxing, and many people use the hot bath, sauna or spa pool as a form of relaxation.

Yoga is a good stretching type of exercise that incorporates some excellent muscle control and relaxation techniques.

Meditation is a powerful form of relaxation, and there is a persuasive body of literature that testifies to its health-promoting benefits.

Relaxation can often be assisted by working through a cassette tape with a programmed relaxation technique. People who have difficulty relaxing on their own sometimes find the use of a biofeedback machine or the assistance of a counsellor can be beneficial.

One of the easiest forms of relaxation is strenuous exercise. This is particularly suitable for the type of person who likes to relax by doing something.

There is often a tendency for the stressed individual to enlist the benefit of drugs (prescription or non-prescription) or alcohol. This is not helpful as it can create a psychological dependence. Nicotine, caffeine and chocolate are all substances that can make relaxation more difficult too. When used habitually they can speed up body metabolism and increase muscle tension.

Relaxation

- A tense muscle can lead to muscle fatigue, with increased tension and pain developing. Learn to consciously relax muscle groups that become tense through overuse or injury.
- An increased state of stress places an additional load on the body and can accelerate muscle and joint fatigue. Incorporate activities into your life that promote relaxation such as yoga, meditation, exercise.
- Avoid the excessive use of stimulants – tea, coffee, tobacco.
- Try and avoid using drugs and alcohol to relax – they can become psychologically addictive.

THE CHRONIC PAIN SUFFERER

I define chronic pain as pain that has been present on a continuous basis for over a year. It tends to produce certain changes that make these cases more complicated and difficult to treat. Hence it requires particular consideration. An acute (short-term) injury is usually limited to one part of the body. A chronic injury tends to cause pain on a more widespread basis. The low back injury can start to cause problems higher up the spine and into the neck. The RSI problem that started in the forearms starts to migrate to the shoulders and neck.

This seems partly due to the body compensating – changing the pattern of use of the body to protect the injured part. This produces a different set of stresses to other parts of the body, which often become symptomatic. It also seems to be related to the nervous system becoming hypersensitive as a result of the chronic and continuous state of excitation of the nerve endings that transmit pain. The nervous system becomes overloaded and small changes can produce an exacerbation of the symptoms. These can include changes in weather, temperature, stress levels and type of activity.

Chronic pain sufferers often have to plan their entire day around what makes them feel better or worse. They may find it difficult to go on long car journeys, sleep in a different bed or engage in unaccustomed physical activity. They often have a disturbed sleep pattern. Pain and the avoidance of it can start to dominate their lives.

It is not always clear what can turn what seems to be an ordinary injury into a chronic one, with a chronic pain pattern. I am sure that there are other lifestyle and personality factors that can contribute to the overloading of the nervous system, where it becomes hypersensitive to pain and other nervous stimuli. When looking at the treatment and management of the chronic pain sufferer it is particularly necessary to take a multifaceted approach to the problem.

- Treat the primary injury and any painful tissues associated with it.
- Treat secondary painful sites and their associated tissues.
- Take a close look at beds, pillows, seating and posture.
- Look at effective self-help measures for both short-term management of pain and long-term management of the condition.
- Look at stress management.
- Therapy is often required for an extended period, as the patient learns to educate him/herself and gain control over the various factors that influence the problem.
- The therapist can act as a signpost, pointing the person in directions that may assist them, and providing information and advice that will assist in their search for the solutions.

Responsibility for the problem is ultimately with the patient, and the exploration for solutions is their challenge. A therapist is a facilitator of this process. It is unlikely that one person can provide this role. Hence the need for a multidisciplinary and multifactorial approach. Look for the pieces of the jigsaw puzzle so that eventually the overall picture becomes clear. Always keep exploring and maintain a positive attitude.

SUMMARY
- Don't ignore early symptoms.
- Treat the symptoms, but pay particular attention to their cause.
- Enlist the support of your employer.
- A doctor or therapist can help in understanding the cause of the problem, assist in finding the solutions, as well as treating the symptoms.
- Take personal responsibility for the problem and learn as much as you can about it.

9

The self-help guide

This chapter details the most common injuries that can be caused, in whole or in part, by our sedentary lifestyles. It gives a guide to the home management of these conditions and the factors that may have contributed to them. The information given is not designed to take the place of professional advice, and this should be sought when appropriate.

The chapter is divided into sections, each dealing with a different region of the body. It outlines the common postural faults that can trigger these problems and some detail about the types of injury. There are diagrams of the common muscular trigger points, followed by a series of exercises that will assist recovery and improve the function of the joints involved.

If you suffer from an area of strain or injury, I recommend a 20 minute daily treatment plan as follows:

- Five minutes' ice therapy.
- Five minutes' trigger point massage.
- Five minutes' ice therapy.
- Five minutes' stretching.

This treatment plan should be performed once a day to the affected area until it becomes symptom free. The recommended exercises should be done in addition once or twice per day. At the end of each section I will also outline the *key exercises*. These are exercises that should be done regularly throughout the day when performing the task that is implicated as a cause of the injury, such as wrist and forearm exercises when keyboarding or low-back exercises when sitting. I generally recommend that this key exercise programme should take about two minutes and should be done hourly while performing the task.

STRETCHING EXERCISES

An overused, fatigued muscle starts to develop stiffness and pain. It develops increased tension putting further stress on the joints and tissues around it. These joints then become mechanically less efficient and a stress–tension–pain cycle develops. The exercises are designed to assist in breaking this cycle, allowing the muscle and its associated joints to work more efficiently.

The initial exercise phase involves stretching the affected muscles around a joint. Once an injury or strain is reduced in intensity and is effectively under control, it may be appropriate to strengthen the muscles to provide better stability and strength to the area. I will detail these exercises where appropriate.

The exercises are very carefully designed to minimise trauma around the joint. There will be times when an injury is too acute to be ready for exercise. In this case continue using ice and massage until the injury has settled sufficiently to begin the exercises.

THE GOLDEN RULE OF EXERCISING
If it hurts – *don't* do it!

An exercise can cause a stretching sensation, but if it actually causes pain do not continue without seeking medical advice first.

The exercise should be performed slowly and held for up to five seconds – *do not* bounce.

ICE THERAPY

This is an important part of the treatment plan and can produce a dramatic improvement in the recovery rate of the tissues. It has the following effects.

- Analgesic – pain reducing.
- Anti-inflammatory.
- Increase in circulation.

The increase in circulation is a secondary effect. On application of the ice the body reduces the circulation to the region in order to preserve body heat. After the ice is removed the body rapidly restores normal temperature by infusing the area with fresh blood. It is this increase in circulation that provides a stimulus to the recuperative powers of the tissues by reducing the amount of swelling, removing some of the products of tissue inflammation and injury, and providing the necessary requirements for tissue regeneration.

There are a number of ways of applying ice therapy and you can choose which is the most convenient.

- A flexible, reusable ice pack.

- Ice cubes wrapped in a damp cloth.
- A bag of frozen peas.
- A frozen, damp tea towel or hand towel, briefly rinsed under cold water to make it more flexible.

The application of moist ice is the most beneficial in its effect, producing a more rapid cooling. Never place something deeply frozen directly onto the skin as this may cause an ice burn. It is better to wrap it in a damp cloth. The ice pack should be placed over the site of injury and the major trigger points around the injury.

With an acute or particularly painful injury the ice packs can be used more frequently throughout the day.

MASSAGE

This can produce a powerful healing effect by assisting relaxation of the muscle fibres. The benefits of massage are described in the previous chapter.

Some areas of the body are accessible to allow self-massage, such as the forearms, while others such as the lumbar spine are best done by a friend. It is possible to self-massage some of the less accessible areas by being a bit creative. For example, lying on top of a tennis ball and using gentle movements until you find the trigger points can be a very good way of massaging the paraspinal muscles. Use some kind of lubricant such as baby oil, vegetable oil or a commercially prepared massage oil. As a general rule massage in the direction of the muscle fibres, paying particular attention to any area that has increased sensitivity or tension. The main trigger points for each region are broadly illustrated, but the exact trigger point can vary from person to person and it is worthwhile to try and identify these. Start with a gentle pressure and gradually become firmer as you progress. It should never be hard enough to cause pain, wincing or a reactive spasm from the muscle you are working on.

If you have had overuse problems in the forearm or hand, the act of massaging could irritate this and so it is best to find someone else to do it, or improvise by using some kind of implement rather than the fingers or thumb. In the kitchen drawer you can probably find something with a smooth, rounded end that would work very well.

Avoid massaging over any open wounds, infected regions or an acutely inflamed injury.

LOW-BACK PAIN

Low-back pain is remarkably common in our society. It is estimated that 80 per cent of the population suffer from low-back pain at some point in their lives. Despite the trend towards mechanisation in our society and the replacement of heavy manual work with sedentary work, the incidence of back problems seems to be increasing. It is my thesis in this book that a significant cause of back pain stems from the evolution of our sedentary lifestyle and the amount of sitting involved.

In less than 20 per cent of cases there is a clear structural cause, such as a disc prolapse or fractured vertebra. In over 80 per cent of cases the problem is more of a functional one with the most obvious symptoms being muscle spasm, joint stiffness and pain.

In approximately 50 per cent of cases the onset is insidious – a gradual onset with no obvious cause. The other 50 per cent are often associated with a particular event, such as lifting or twisting. These are often relatively insignificant and it is reasonable to suggest there are other factors involved.

I believe that the compression of the spine caused by prolonged sitting renders the spine much more liable to injury from relatively minor strains. In 1991 in the UK, there were over 67 million working days lost through back injuries at an estimated cost to society of over £3 billion.

Associated causes

- Stiffness in the spinal joints and hips.
- Tight hamstrings.
- Weak abdominal muscles.
- Poor sitting posture – a faulty chair
  - a low flat desk
  - inadequate back support
  - leaning too far forward.
- Poor bending/lifting technique.

A simple back strain will usually respond to treatment promptly, but there is a high incidence of recurrent episodes. A chronic injury with damage or deterioration of the spine will require extra care and management.

Trigger points

These commonly occur at the following sites:

- At the levels of the affected vertebrae, either side of the spine.
- Between the spine and pelvis.
- The gluteal muscles at the buttocks.

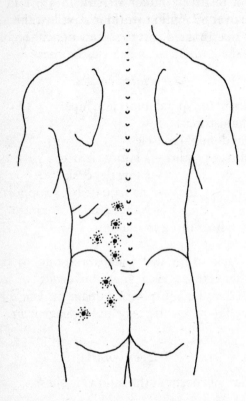

Pain from the low back will often refer into the hip/gluteal or groin regions and sometimes down the leg. In some cases involvement of the sciatic nerve can cause severe leg pain.

Flexibility exercises for the low back

Knee hugging

Gently pull the knee toward the chest. Hold for five seconds, then relax. Repeat five times each leg. A variation is to pull the knee up to and across the chest.

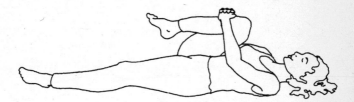

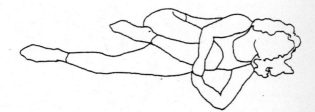

Back extension

Lying on your front with the weight on the elbows allows a gentle traction on the spine after long periods of sitting. Hold for up to 10 minutes. A gentle extension stretch can be performed by straightening the arms.

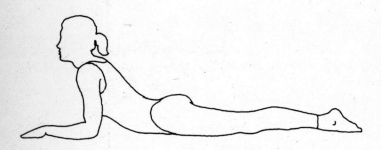

Side bending

While leaning side-on against a wall with your arm slightly bent, allow your pelvis to gently drop towards the wall. Repeat up to 10 times each side.

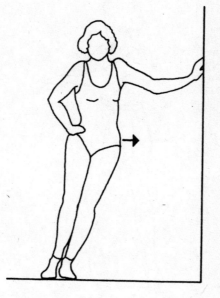

Standing twist

With feet about 15 inches apart, use the weight of the arms to rotate your torso gently. Develop a rhythmic movement for 20 to 30 seconds.

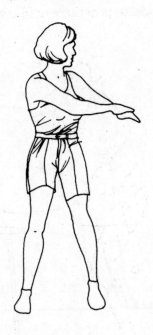

Hamstring stretch

See chapter 4 for information about hamstrings and how to test them.

- Place heel with straight leg on a raised surface. Keeping your back straight, bend the supporting leg. Hold for five seconds. Repeat three to four times for each leg.

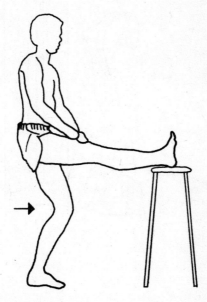

- Lying on your back, place a leg straight up against the wall until hamstrings are stretched. Hold for 20 to 30 seconds for each leg. This is a good position for an isometric contraction, followed by stretch (see chapter 8).

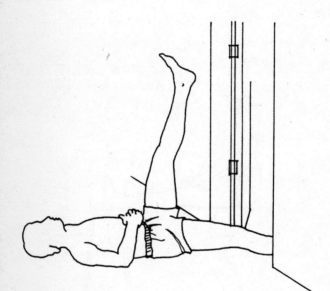

Iliopsoas stretch

See chapter 4 for information about iliopsoas. Place one foot flat on the floor, while kneeling on the other leg. Lean forward at the knee and backward at the waist. Hold for five seconds, repeat three to four times each side.

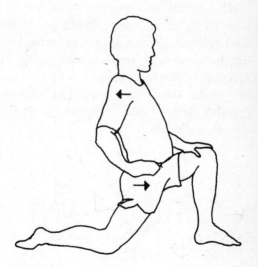

Key exercises

- Side bending.
- Standing twist.

Strengthening exercises for the low back

Abdominal curl – stomach muscles

Lying on your back, knees bent, arms folded across chest, lift your head and shoulders until shoulderblades are just off the floor, but low back remains supported. Hold for three to five seconds. Repeat 10 times.

Variation: while sitting up, twist so elbow moves towards opposite knee. Hold for three to five seconds. Repeat five times each side.

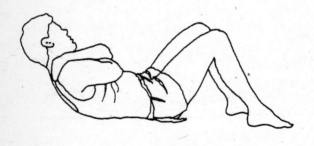

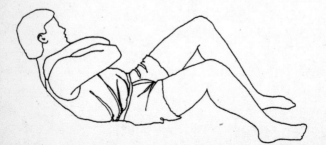

Be careful. It is very easy to do this exercise wrong, and it is often the cause of injury.

- Always have knees up.
- Keep arms folded across chest (not behind neck or head).
- Keep lumbar spine supported on the floor.
- Keep eyes fixed on ceiling (do not overstrain neck).

Spinal extensions

Lying on your stomach, arms by your side, slightly raise your head and shoulders off the floor while raising one leg. Hold for five seconds. Repeat five times for each leg, then five times while raising both legs.

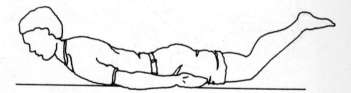

Pelvic curls

Lying on your back, with the knees bent and arms by side, do the following simultaneously:

- Suck tummy in.
- Tilt the pelvis forward.
- Squeeze the buttocks together.

Hold for five seconds. Repeat 10 times.

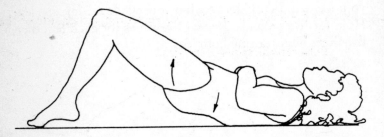

MID-BACK PAIN

This is where pain or discomfort occurs in the middle section of the spine, approximately from the bottom of the ribs to the middle of the shoulderblades. It very commonly occurs as a secondary pain area with either a low-back injury or a neck and shoulder strain. It can also occur as a primary strain; these are usually caused by awkward twisting movements or a slouched posture.

Associated causes

- Stiffness in spinal joints and hips.
- Tight hamstrings.
- Weak abdominal muscles.
- Poor sitting posture – a poor chair
  – a low flat desk
  – leaning too far forward
  – slouching.
- An awkward or repeated twisting posture.

Trigger points

- At the levels of the affected vertebrae, either side of the spine.
- Between the shoulderblades.

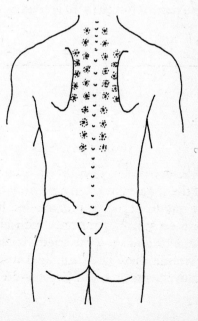

Flexibility exercises for the mid-back

Most of the exercises that assist the flexibility of the mid-back have been described in the low-back section, with the addition of the sitting twist.

- Back extension.
- Side bending.
- Standing twist.
- Sitting twist (see below).

Sitting twist

Sit backwards on a fixed chair. Clasp your fingers together in front, holding elbows outstretched. Rotate your head and trunk from side to side, leading with elbows. Develop a rhythmic movement for 20 to 30 seconds.

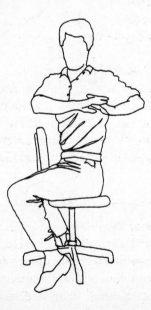

There is an association with mid-back pain and hamstring stiffness. If either psoas or hamstring muscles are tight, these should also be stretched.

Key exercises

- Side bending.
- Standing twist.
- Sitting twist.

Strengthening exercises for the mid-back

These have been described in the low-back section with the addition of the modified standing twist. Those recommended are:

- Abdominal curl.
- Spinal extensions.
- Modified standing twist.

Modified standing twist

The standing twist, as described in the flexibility exercises for the low back, is modified with the addition of a weight in each hand. Start with 500gm, building up to 1kg. This should be done for 30 seconds, gradually building up to two minutes. This provides strength and flexibility.

Neck and shoulder pain

The neck is the most flexible part of the spine. It is also required to support the weight of the head. In the working situation the head and neck are manoeuvred into positions that allow effective vision. Movements of the neck involve quite specific groups of small strap-like muscles which can easily become fatigued when required to work for long periods of time. Some of these muscles, such as the upper trapezius and levator scapula, come down the neck and join onto the shoulderblades.

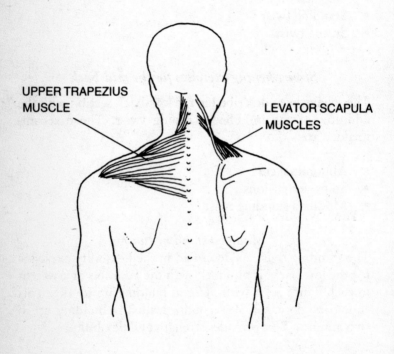

UPPER TRAPEZIUS MUSCLE

LEVATOR SCAPULA MUSCLES

These muscles are probably the most common source of trigger points in the body and are a frequent source of neck and shoulder pain and headaches. It is via these muscles that the positioning of the arms and shoulderblades can be major factors in creating neck tension.

The neck functions best when able to work in an upright position close to its centre of gravity. The further it departs from this the greater the likelihood of developing muscle strains. The shoulderblades develop least strain when the arms are able to relax hanging loosely by the side of the body without elevation of the shoulders.

Associated causes

Poor neck and head position:

- Poor visual angle – work too low.
- Continually looking to one side – poor position of screen, work or copy holder.
- Visual difficulty – work too far away
  - incorrect glasses
  - glare or reflection
  - screen poorly adjusted.

Poor shoulder position:

- Work surface or keyboard too high.
- Over-reaching – work too far away.
- Inadequate wrist or forearm support.
- Stress – difficulty relaxing.
- Carrying heavy bags.

Trigger points

Poor neck and head position:

- Suboccipital muscles – the muscles that attach the back of the skull to the top of the neck.
- Trapezius muscle and muscles at the back of the neck.
- Between the shoulderblades.

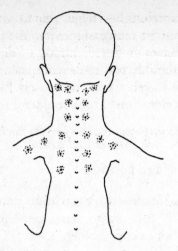

Poor shoulder position:

- At the back of the neck.
- On top of the shoulderblades.
- Between the shoulderblades.

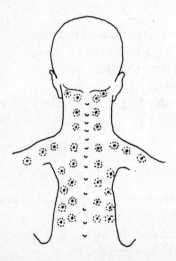

For the person who enjoys trigger point massage this is a fertile area! There are many trigger points to be located in these hard-working muscles. Massage can be of great benefit to ease tension and reduce stress for problems in this region.

Flexibility exercises for the neck

Rotation

Gently rotate the neck to one side as far as it will comfortably go. Hold for three seconds. Repeat five times each side.

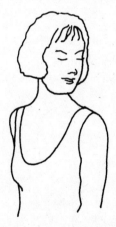

Side bending

Keeping the chin in the midline, gently side bend the neck as far as it will comfortably go. Hold for three seconds. Repeat five times each side.

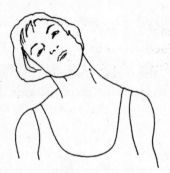

Neck rolls

In the side-bent position, as in the previous exercise, gently move the head and neck forwards as far as it will comfortably go, hold for two seconds, then backwards, hold for two seconds. Repeat five times each side. Remember:

- Keep chin in the midline.
- Keep shoulders relaxed.
- Avoid extremes of forward and backward bending in the neck.

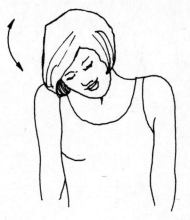

Shoulder shrugging

Raise the shoulders up toward the ears. Hold for three seconds, then rapidly let them relax. Repeat five times (see page 168, chapter 8 for a full explanation of this exercise).

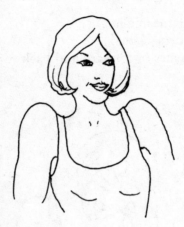

Flexibility exercises for the shoulderblades

Rotation

With the arms hanging loosely by the side, rotate the shoulders forwards in as large a circle as possible, in one rhythmic movement. Repeat five times forward, five times backward.

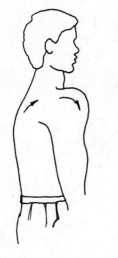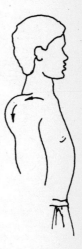

Forward stretch

With arms held in front, back of hands together, and thumbs pointing to the floor, reach forward with the arms as far as possible. Hold for three seconds. Repeat five times.

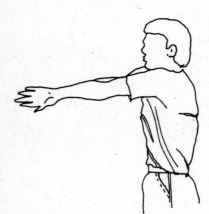

Backward stretch

With arms behind the back, palms together and fingers interlaced, stretch backwards with the arms as far as possible. Hold for three seconds. Repeat five times.

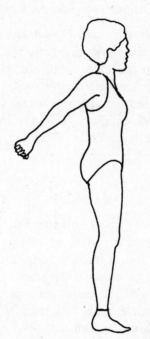

Key exercises

* Rotation.
* Side bending.
* Shoulder rotations.

Strengthening exercises for the neck and shoulders.

The muscles involved in this region are mainly postural muscles and are active under most circumstances. They are unlikely to develop specific weaknesses. However, there is evidence that suggests the stronger these muscles are, the less effort is required for postural work, which leads to a reduction in the risk of injury. The exercise par excellence for strengthening this region is swimming. A well-designed gym programme can be helpful.

HEADACHES

Headaches are a very common feature of our modern life. They can come from a variety of causes. They are often related to an infection. A fever or sinus infection will cause a temporary headache which disappears when the infection clears. Pressure inside the brain, such as that caused by a tumour, is very rare and will usually produce other neurological symptoms as well.

Most headaches do not have a readily identifiable cause – these tend to be described as tension headaches. They often start at the back of the head or top of the neck and as they progress they move forward to above or behind the eyes and the temples. Some researchers have estimated that 90 per cent of headaches are caused by neck tension. The neck tension is usually produced by poor posture, with the small strap-like neck muscles often being required to hold the head in a forward-bent position for long periods of time. The muscles involved are usually the suboccipital muscles and the muscles between the neck and shoulders such as trapezius and levator scapular. These muscles will feel tight and ropey with tender trigger points.

The pattern of pain will usually show that the pain gets worse throughout the day as the working or studying posture builds up tension. It can remain quite severe in the evenings, but is usually better at weekends or days off. It is usually better after a good night's sleep, provided you have a comfortable sleeping position and a good pillow. Tension headaches can be chronic, severe and very debilitating, and often produce a type of depression. Fortunately they tend to respond rapidly to manual therapy. Most patients who arrive for treatment with a headache are able to leave without one.

The self-treatment for tension headaches follows that described for neck tension, with the exercises and trigger points being very valuable methods of self-help. To prevent further episodes of these tension headaches, take a very careful look at your sitting posture, particularly the neck and head position, and follow the ergonomic advice described in this book.

The migraine is a particular type of headache that seems to be caused by spasm and dilation of the blood vessels to the brain. There is often a hereditary tendency to have migraine. It produces a severe headache of sudden onset, often accompanied by nausea, vomiting and visual disturbances. Migraines can have a variety of triggers, such as stress, muscle tension, food (cheese, chocolate and alcohol are common) or hormonal factors. The differentiation between tension headaches and migraine is a blurry one, with many cases of tension headaches misdiagnosed as migraine. Many migraine sufferers also get tension headaches and get considerable benefit from a treatment programme as described here.

A severe headache occurring with high fever and a stiff neck is suggestive of meningitis. This requires urgent medical attention.

PILLOWS

Anybody suffering from neck tension or headaches should have the best pillow available. Sleeping is an opportunity for the muscles to relax completely and restore normal function. You should wake up in the morning feeling better than when you went to sleep. If this is not the case take a close look at your sleeping posture.

Most people like to sleep on their side, they usually go to sleep on one side and then vary sides throughout the night. The requirement for a pillow here is to fill the space between your shoulder and neck, allowing your neck and head to follow a continuous straight line with the rest of your spine.

Sleeping flat on your tummy is not a good idea. It twists the neck into an awkward position and is associated with increased levels of neck tension. If you have to sleep on your tummy it is better to have no pillow at all, or at least a very thin one. The recovery position (a mixture of front and side) is a better one.

Some people like to sleep on their backs, and here the pillow is required to keep the head and neck following the natural spinal curves, similar to standing.

Look for a pillow that moulds to the contours of your body shape and at the same time provides relaxation and support. I usually recommend a mixture of feather and down as being the best, and foam rubber or foam chip as the worst. The density of the pillow required depends on the body shape and the sleeping position adopted.

THE SHOULDER AND UPPER ARM

This section relates to the shoulder joint proper, i.e. the joint between the arm and the shoulderblade, and the muscles that envelop it. It is structured a little differently from some of the other joints and this structure allows it added flexibility – it is the loosest joint in the body. Most joints have strong ligaments that surround them, limiting their movement and providing stability. In place of a strong ligamentous structure, the shoulder joint has a 'nest' of muscles known as the rotator cuff. This nest of muscles allows added flexibility and good control at the shoulder in many different positions. These muscles are relatively small compared to the large forces that can develop when the arm is used at a distance from the body. As a result these muscles are easily prone to injury.

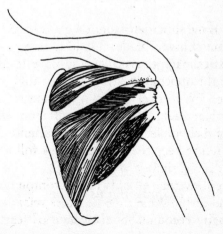

Fig. 9.1 The rotator cuff muscles of the shoulder.

The injuries are caused by:

- Manipulating objects at a distance.
- Working in an awkward position.
- Holding the arm away from the body for long periods of time.

In the sitting posture the factors most likely to cause shoulder strain are:

- Work surface or keyboard too high.
- Work surface or keyboard too far away.
- Continual awkward reaching movements, particularly overhead or behind.

Trigger points for the shoulder

The trigger points are located at the site of the rotator cuff muscles (see illustration on page 207):

- On top of the shoulderblade.
- Behind the shoulderblade.
- Outside of the upper arm.
- Front of the upper arm.

It is worthwhile going into more detail about some of the most common shoulder strains and the approach to treating them.

Supraspinatus strain

This is the most common shoulder injury. It can be caused by a fall on the shoulder or outstretched arm. It is commonly caused by overuse of the arm away from the side of the body or by carrying heavy bags. It causes pain around the point of the shoulder and the outside of the upper arm. The pain is usually felt on shoulder movement of the arm away from the body, often with a noticeable clicking. The pain increases until the arm is past the horizontal and then eases as it rises above the shoulder. This is known as a painful arc of motion and is characteristic of the supraspinatous strain. It often causes pain at night and patients complain of not being able to sleep on that shoulder. It responds well to trigger point treatment and exercises. The trigger points are beneath the trapezius muscle and require deep pressure.

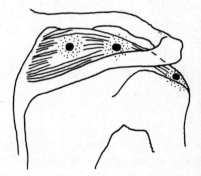

Anterior shoulder strain

There are two muscles that work together at the front of the shoulder and are commonly strained: the anterior portion of the deltoid muscle and the long head of the biceps muscle.

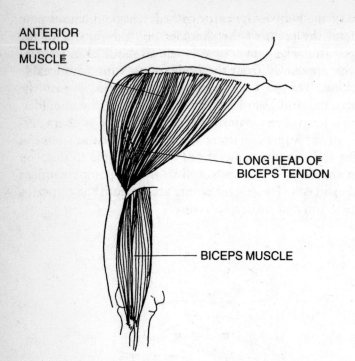

ANTERIOR
DELTOID
MUSCLE

LONG HEAD OF
BICEPS TENDON

BICEPS MUSCLE

The deltoid is the large muscle overlaying the shoulder joint forming the shape of the upper arm. It is the front portion of this muscle that becomes involved. The biceps muscle is an important muscle at the front of the arm involved in many shoulder and elbow movements. The long head of biceps is a tendon from this muscle that crosses the bony surface of the shoulder joint and is often required to work at an awkward angle.

The pain from these muscles is felt at the front of the shoulder, and tends to be aggravated by raising the arm in front of the body or across the chest. It is commonly subject to strain with a faulty working position. It is also often injured by racquet sports, particularly with forehand or overhead shots. This area responds well to treatment with ice and trigger point massage, but care should be taken to isolate and avoid the irritating movements.

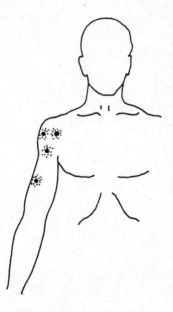

Flexibility exercises for the shoulder

Forward stretch

See flexibility exercises for the shoulderblades (pages 201–3).

Backward stretch

See flexibility exercises for the shoulderblades (pages 201–3).

Doorway stretch

With the forearms supported either side of a doorway and one leg in front of the other, gradually lean forward while bending the front knee. Hold this stretch for five seconds. Repeat five times.

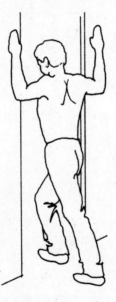

Across body stretch

With the arm across the body and forearm over the opposite shoulder, use the other hand to pull on the elbow. Hold for five seconds. Repeat five times.

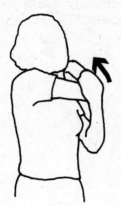

Behind head stretch

With the arm over and behind the head, use the other hand to gently pull back on the elbow. Hold for five seconds. Repeat five times.

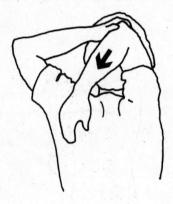

Behind back stretch

With one arm behind the head reaching between shoulder-blades, bring other arm behind the back to meet and clasp fingers. If you cannot reach, use a tea towel or belt suspended from your top hand to pull the hands together gently. Hold for 30 seconds. Repeat with arms reversed.

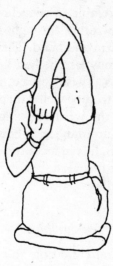

Key exercises

- Backward stretch.
- Across body stretch.
- Behind head stretch.

Shoulder strengthening exercises

Swimming, gym workouts, martial arts, such as kung fu or T'ai Chi.

ELBOW AND FOREARM PAIN

The elbow is a strong, stable joint. It is known as a hinge joint because it operates in one plane of movement. In addition to the elbow being able to bend and straighten, the two forearm bones are able to swivel around each other, allowing the hand to rotate through 180°, giving more flexibility to the forearm and hand. The elbow is operated by strong, well-sited muscles, the best known of which are the biceps and triceps. These can be injured by forceful movements, but seem to cope well with postural stress. The muscles that operate the wrist and fingers extend up the forearm and attach around the elbow. These are very common sites of strain. It is in fact the position of the wrist and the movements at the wrist, hands and fingers that are responsible for most elbow pain.

Tennis elbow

This is a very common condition and can be caused by many activities rather than just tennis. It is most commonly caused by repetitive type strains and perhaps is the most classic of the RSIs. It usually starts in the dominant arm, but can spread to both. It starts with a dull aching on the outside of the elbow, which is aggravated by gripping with the hand, twisting or backward bending the wrist. Some movements, such as picking up a kettle or opening a jar, can cause a sudden pain, causing the arm to go weak and occasionally drop things. It is caused by an overstrain at the wrist extensor (backward bending) muscles, and its common medical name is extensor tendonitis.

This group of extensor muscles join together to form a common insertion on the outside of the elbow. This is a fairly small attachment for a powerful group of muscles that often work continuously throughout the day. The insertion can be easily strained through overuse and can become a very hot trigger point.

There are usually other trigger points in the forearm depending on which actions have been straining particular muscles. These muscles have slightly differing actions according to their role. Some extend just the wrist, some extend the fingers or thumb, and others are more concerned with the twisting movement of the forearm. Try and isolate which action causes the pain and then work your way up the forearm until you find the muscles involved and their trigger points. With a little bit of searching they can be accurately located. It is well worth making the effort as these muscles respond very well to trigger point massage.

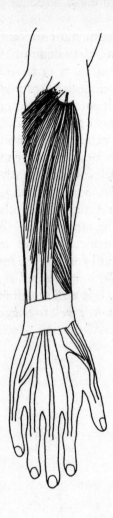

Fig. 9.2 The wrist extensor muscles of the forearm.

It is also necessary to try and reduce the workload on the affected area by avoiding the strain-provoking action and improving the ergonomics of the working position. The most common actions that cause tennis elbow are:

- Manual work: using a screwdriver, hammering, using pruning shears, pliers, etc.
- Backhand shots with racquet sports.
- Writer's cramp – tight gripping of a pen.
- Typing and keyboard work – particularly if the keyboard is too high, producing an extended wrist posture.
- Absence of effective wrist support can also be a factor.

Golfer's elbow

This is less common than tennis elbow and occurs on the inside of the elbow and forearm. This involves the flexor group (forward bending) muscles of the wrist and hand and is medically known as flexor tendonitis. The type of pain and mechanism of onset is very similar to tennis elbow. It is generally caused by tight gripping and flexion movements of the wrist. The most common trigger point is at the attachment of the muscles on the inside of the elbow. There are usually other trigger points in the group of muscles associated with wrist and finger flexion on the underside of the forearm.

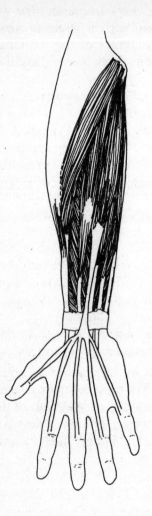

Fig. 9.3 The wrist flexor muscles of the forearm.

This can be caused by movements that bend the wrist forward, particularly with a gripping action. Common causative factors are:

- The golf swing.
- Forearm shots with racquet sports.
- Forward bent wrist – the left-handed writer or a poor keyboard position.

Both these conditions respond very well to the treatment programme as described at the beginning of the chapter. In addition to the ice–massage–exercise sequence, relative rest is important. This requires avoiding the action that produced the strain or improving the ergonomics of it. In some cases there are benefits from wearing a tight, non-elastic band just below the elbow when the wrist and forearm are being used extensively. This reduces the amount of stress at the muscle insertions, while still allowing good muscle activity.

The recommended exercises for this condition will be shown at the end of the following section dealing with the wrist and hand.

WRIST AND HAND PAIN

Tendonitis

Tendonitis is a very common finding in the tendons of the muscles that produce wrist flexion and extension. The illustrations on pages 218 and 220 show how the lower arm muscles form tendons just before they cross the wrist. The tendons attach to various parts of the wrist or hand. Tendonitis is an inflammation of the tendon or its sheath. It characteristically causes an aching pain on or after use of the muscle and its tendon. This pain can be provoked by a strong movement of the wrist while clenching the fist. There is usually a noticeable swelling of the tendon which becomes quite sore to touch.

Tendonitis is usually caused by overuse – repetitive movements of the hand and wrist. These repetitive movements are more stressful when the wrist is used outside its comfort zone or is combined with a forceful gripping action.

It is very common on production lines with jobs that require frequent repetition. It is widely recognised to be a common disorder associated with typing and VDU work. The common causative factors are:

- Overuse.
- Poor keyboard height and position.
- Inadequate wrist support.
- Poor wrist posture.

The problem is often aggravated by increasing stiffness and muscle tension developing in the wrist joint and forearm muscles. This condition responds very well to ice, massage and a stretching programme. As well as the inflamed tendon, there will be trigger points in the associated muscles in the forearm. These must also be massaged and released. Careful consideration should be given to the angle at which the wrist is being used.

Ganglion

A ganglion is a small fluid-filled cyst, usually found on the back of the hand or wrist. It communicates with a tendon or joint capsule and usually arises spontaneously. Some authorities associate it with overuse. It varies in size somewhere between a pea and a marble and can become very hard resembling bone. It can be slightly tender, but is usually pain free. Ganglions frequently disappear spontaneously, but if they are troublesome they can be surgically excised.

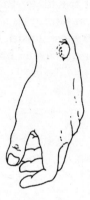

Fig. 9.4 A ganglion on the wrist.

De Quervain's disease

This is a sinister-sounding name for an inflammation of the tendons at the base of the thumb. These can easily be found by bending the thumb backwards. This makes the tendons prominent, creating a small hollow between them known as the anatomical snuff box. It is usually caused by prolonged gripping with the thumb and repetitive movements involving backward and sideways bending of the wrist. Treat the trigger points in the tendon and its muscle and look closely at the action that is causing it.

Trigger finger

Trigger finger is a snapping sensation of the finger during bending and straightening. It is caused by a nodule forming in the flexor tendon of the finger that prevents a smooth movement of the tendon within its sheath. The finger can become stuck in a trigger position and can only be straightened out by using the other hand.

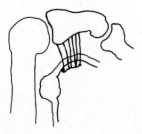

Fig. 9.5 A swelling in the tendon can cause trigger finger.

It is usually caused by overuse producing a tendonitis. To treat this problem, discover and avoid the action that initiated the problem. It will often settle with the use of massage and the passing of time. If it remains a problem, a cortisone injection is usually successful. It occasionally affects the thumb.

Carpal tunnel syndrome

This is a common disorder caused by an entrapment of the median nerve at the carpal tunnel which is found on the underside of the wrist. It commonly affects middle-aged females in one or both hands. It is also common during pregnancy. The compression of the nerve is usually caused by a tendonitis of the flexor tendons, with subsequent swelling causing pressure on the median nerve. It usually causes pain and tingling in the first three fingers and sometimes in the forearm. The discomfort is usually worse at night. If it becomes advanced it can cause weakness and numbness in the fingers, making it difficult to pick up small objects. The pain can often be brought on or aggravated by bending the wrist forward or backward.

It is usually regarded as an overuse injury brought on by repeated gripping with the hand and forward bending of the wrist. It is often related to fluid retention, such as in pregnancy, using oral contraceptives or premenstrual tension. If it is recognised early, it can usually be relieved by isolating and avoiding the movements that aggravate it; massaging and stretching the flexor tendons and muscles; and exercises to mobilise the wrist. A wrist support or splint to keep the wrist in a neutral position while working can be helpful. If fluid retention is a factor, this should be addressed. In more advanced cases cortisone injection or surgery may be necessary.

Flexibility exercises for the forearm, wrist and hand

The prayer
With the hands held in front in the prayer position, raise the elbows as high as is comfortable. Hold for five seconds. Then, keeping the fingers together and spread, separate the

palms and raise the elbows as high as is comfortable.
Repeat both stages three times.

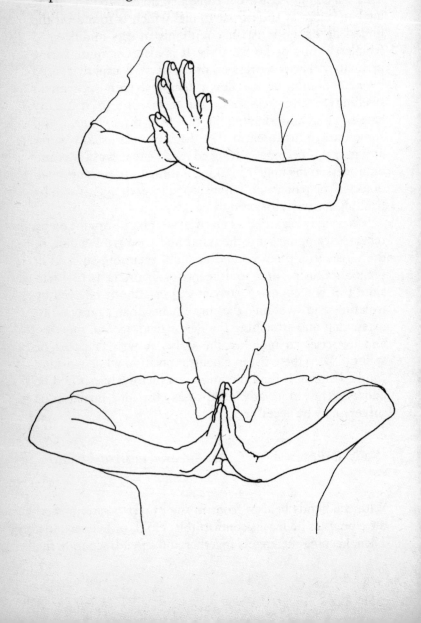

Wrist extensor stretch

With one arm outstretched use the other hand to bend the wrist, hand and fingers fully forward. Hold for five seconds. Repeat three times for each arm.

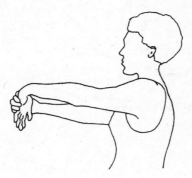

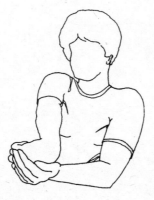

Wrist rotations

Rotate the hand and wrist in as wide a circle as possible. Repeat five times clockwise and anti-clockwise with each hand.

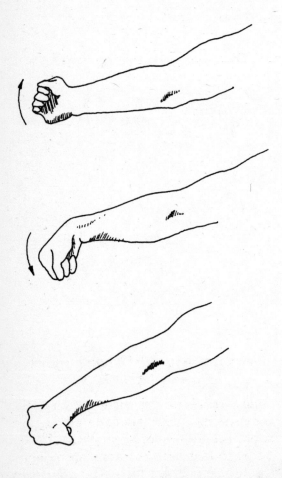

Shake it all about!

With the hands and fingers relaxed, use the rest of the arm to shake the wrist. Try and develop up and down and side to side shaking. Do both hands together for about 15 seconds.

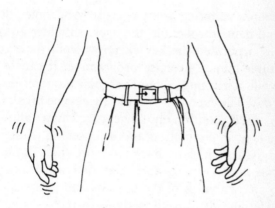

Key exercises

All of them!

Strengthening exercises for the forearm, wrist and hand

Strengthening exercises for this region are very valuable in reducing the stress and rate of fatigue during continued use. It can help prevent future overuse problems. The exercises should not be started until the arms are symptom free (without professional advice first). The exercises usually involve squeezing or gripping or repeated wrist movements while holding some form of weight. It is difficult to provide a recommended exercise regime that would suit everyone. If you have had problems in the forearms or hands I would suggest that you seek professional advice as to the type and intensity of exercises that would be appropriate for you.

THE THREE-MINUTE UPPER BODY STRETCH

Most people suffering from overuse syndromes develop aches and pains throughout the neck, shoulder and arms. I have incorporated the key exercises from these regions into a three-minute exercise programme. It can be done easily while remaining seated at regular intervals throughout the day. The exercises provide a welcome break for the muscles used continually. The stretching allows an improvement in circulation and a loosening of the joints and soft tissues which both lead to more efficient functioning. Doing these exercises at regular intervals allows you to develop an awareness of the muscles and joints and their state of fatigue. It also allows you to recognise areas of dysfunction before they become serious. With practice the exercises as listed take between two and two and a half minutes, which allows for you to spend a little extra time on the ones that are most important for you.

THE THREE-MINUTE UPPER BODY STRETCH

- Sitting twist – five times each side (page 192).
- Backward shoulder stretch – hold for 10 seconds (page 203).
- Shoulder rotations – both shoulders five times clockwise and anti-clockwise (page 201).
- Across body shoulder stretch – five seconds each shoulder (page 213).

- Neck rotations – hold three seconds, twice each side (page 197).
- Neck roll – 10 seconds each side (page 199).
- Prayer position – each stage for five seconds each (page 225).
- Wrist extensor stretch – 10 seconds each arm (page 227).
- Wrist shaking – both hands for 10 seconds (page 229).

10

Fit for life

BENEFITS OF EXERCISE

Exercise is a wonderful panacea. It stimulates the mind, invigorates the body and benefits the psyche. There are many well-documented health benefits from exercise. Regular aerobic exercise significantly reduces the incidence of heart attacks, strokes, atherosclerosis and other circulatory problems. It has a normalising effect in cases of high or low blood pressure. Exercise has a hormone balancing effect, and can help regulate hormone cycles during menopause or premenstrual problems. It has a powerful antidepressive effect and can help reduce stress levels. It helps boost energy levels and concentration. It helps reduce the risk of injury by improving muscle tone. It uses up calories and can help to normalise weight levels. It is a powerful antidote to the health problems created by our stressful but physically sedentary lifestyles.

If this isn't enough to convince you that regular exercise should be a part of your life, then perhaps you should know that there is good evidence that people who exercise regularly have an improved sex life!

All these wonderful health-giving benefits from something that need cost very little. You often hear people lament the lack of time for regular exercise. I believe that exercising regularly creates its own time. The improved functioning, better concentration and reduction in fatigue produced by regular exercise more than compensates for the time taken.

STARTING AN EXERCISE PROGRAMME

Be careful! The easiest time to get injured is in the early stages of exercising when enthusiasm is greater than the capacity to perform. Always warm up first, do a few appropriate stretching exercises before commencing.

If you haven't exercised for a while, start gently, do not push yourself until your body has had a chance to adapt to this new pursuit. The body is capable of performing the most demanding endeavours, but it needs time to adjust. Twice a week is often enough when beginning as it can take at least three days to recover in the early stages. After a month you can think about increasing the frequency. There is an old runner's adage – never to increase your mileage by more than 10 per cent a week. To do more than that invites the risk of injury. This applies equally to other forms of exercise.

The first month can seem rather painful, like hard work, until your body becomes tuned in to this new pursuit and develops an easy rhythm. Persevere for that first month because it will soon become pleasurable. It is often helpful to join in with other people or clubs and benefit from the dynamics of a group activity.

SOME TYPES OF EXERCISE

Swimming

This is a very good exercise to start with or when rehabilitating from an injury as the relatively weightless environment gives a low injury risk, while benefiting both upper and lower body and improving cardiovascular fitness.

Freestyle is the preferred stroke, and it is important to breathe on both sides as this allows the body to function in a good balance. Breaststroke can be a strain on the neck and the inside of the knees. For every two lengths of freestyle it is a good idea to do one of backstroke as this aids muscle balance. If you are unused to swimming or have difficulty with breathing or other techniques, a little bit of coaching in the early stages can be very helpful.

'Aquarobics' and 'aquacise' exercise classes in water are excellent forms of exercise.

Cycling

This is an excellent form of exercise that doubles as a very good, ecologically friendly form of transport. Make sure the seat is set at the right height and that you don't have to overstretch to reach the handlebars. For long cycle rides it is a good idea to have a variety of handlebar grips to help reduce any postural stresses.

Jogging

This is one of the quickest methods of gaining the benefits of exercise but can be quite hard on the joints. Good running shoes make a big difference, as does trying to avoid continually running on hard surfaces such as roads or concrete. Avoid bad road cambers. Running often receives bad publicity, but if done sensibly it is an excellent way to improve health and fitness.

Walking

This is excellent exercise that can be done at any age. It can be started at a very gentle level, and brisk walking is nearly as beneficial as running while avoiding the risk of injuries. It is an ideal introduction to exercising that can be tailored to suit any age group or fitness level.

Gym workouts

There are excellent exercise programmes that can be specifically tailored for your requirements. Most exercise stations are well designed, with the body well supported. Make sure that the gym instructors are well qualified and able to advise on particular exercises that will benefit you and any that you should avoid. Ensure the gym is well supervised.

Exercise classes

These can vary from the excellent to the hazardous. It all depends on the type of programme, the degree of fitness and the quality of instruction. Always choose the gentle routines when beginning and ensure the instructor is well qualified.

SOUND NUTRITION

Sensible eating is an important requirement for optimum health. Our sedentary lifestyles, with the high proportion of sitting involved, predisposes us towards certain health problems. Sound nutrition enables us to minimise the negative effects of the relatively inactive lives we lead. Some of the principles of good nutrition that apply to our sedentary lifestyles are outlined below.

Calories

Sitting doesn't use up many calories and it becomes very easy to gain weight by consuming more calories than you are able to burn off. Regular exercise is helpful in counteracting this effect.

It is also good practice to balance the diet in favour of low-calorie foods such as fruit, salad, vegetables and wholegrains. The foods with the highest calorie content are foods with a high proportion of fat (meat, cheese, fried foods, etc.) and refined carbohydrate (white flour and sugar). These should be restricted.

Fat

Our typical Western diet has a high proportion of fat. As well as fat's high calorie content providing a tendency toward obesity, it is linked to circulatory problems, such as atherosclerosis (hardening of the arteries) and heart disease. Long periods of inactivity, such as sitting and a generally sedentary lifestyle, are important predisposing factors in developing a build up of fatty deposits in the arteries. Exercise is protective against heart disease, whereas a lack of exercise promotes it. A diet low in saturated fats is protective against artery disease. Some sources of fat can be protective against heart disease. These are principally vegetable and fish oils.

Carbohydrates

Some researchers have found a connection between fatigue in the workplace and blood-sugar levels. Concentration and performance are reduced with low blood-sugar and there is a higher rate of errors and accidents as a result. It is sensible to keep blood-sugar levels stable throughout the day. It is important not to skip breakfast and to plan healthy snacks for long periods between meals. Foods high in refined carbohydrate generally produce a rapid increase in blood-sugar levels, which can be followed by a rebound effect producing low blood-sugar. For good health and stable blood-sugar levels unrefined carbohydrates (wholemeal products) with minimal sugar levels are preferable.

Roughage (fibre)

Long periods of sitting lead to sluggish bowel function. This can lead to constipation, diverticulitis and other bowel problems. A number of researchers have shown an increased incidence of cancer of the bowel in sedentary workers. A diet high in roughage improves bowel function and is protective against bowel cancer. Fibre is found in fruit, vegetables and wholegrains.

SUMMARY

Sensible eating patterns for a sedentary lifestyle include:

- Low fat – restrict meat, dairy foods, fried foods – encourage fish and white meats.
- Low calorie and high fibre – encourage fruit, vegetables and grains.
- Complex carbohydrate – avoid sugar and refined flour products – encourage wholemeal foods, grains, seeds, fruit and vegetables.

Vitamins and minerals

Good nutrition is an essential requirement for good health. Adequate levels of vitamins and minerals are necessary for healthy functioning of the body. Some nutrients are of special concern when considering muscle pain and fatigue. These are:

- Vitamins – B1, B6, B12, folic acid, vitamin C.
- Minerals – calcium, iron, potassium, magnesium.

Deficiency of these nutritional factors is commonly associated with musculoskeletal problems, and it is important to ensure a good dietary intake. Supplements of these vitamins and minerals can be helpful in improving recovery from muscle and joint problems if any of the deficiency symptoms are present. Most vitamins and minerals require co-factors for efficient absorption and effective functioning. For this reason supplements should always be taken with meals. Examples of co-factors are: iron absorption can be increased by the presence of vitamin C; vitamins A and D are necessary

for the absorption of calcium. Depletion of vitamins and
minerals can commonly occur due to:

- Poor diet.
- Inadequate absorption.
- Additional requirements.

Our modern diet with its emphasis on refined, processed
and stored foods can lead to inadequate levels of some
nutritional factors. Some nutrients are difficult to absorb,
such as iron and calcium, and have to be taken in amounts
greater than that required by the body.

The amount of particular vitamins and minerals required
can vary from person to person. This is known as bio-
chemical individuality. Other lifestyle and health factors can
increase requirements of certain nutrients. For example:

- Excess bleeding during menstruation can lead to iron
  deficiency.
- Early menopause can increase calcium requirements.
- Smoking, stress, excess alcohol consumption and using
  oral contraceptives are known to increase requirements
  of particular vitamins.

I will briefly outline the important nutritional requirements
for musculoskeletal health.

Vitamin B1

- Function – required for efficient function of nerves and
  muscles.
- Deficiency symptoms – calf cramps at night, fluid
  retention, constipation, fatigue, depression and muscle
  weakness.

- Causes of deficiency – junk food diet, high alcohol intake, pregnancy, stress.
- Sources – wholegrains and rice.

Vitamin B6

- Function – essential for proper function of brain, hormones and muscles.
- Deficiency symptoms – acne, depression, irritability, premenstrual fluid retention.
- Causes of deficiency – dieting, contraceptive pill, pregnancy, diabetes, poor diet, alcohol, smoking.
- Sources – grains, nuts, yeast, bananas, rice.

Vitamin B12

- Function – necessary for digestion of protein and good nerve and cell function.
- Deficiency symptoms – can lead to pernicious anaemia: exhaustion, pale skin, breathlessness, numbness, tingling in hands and feet, difficulty walking, confusion.
- Causes of deficiency – vegetarianism, old age (poor diet), heavy drinking or smoking.
- Sources – animal and dairy products.

Folic acid

- Function – necessary for a healthy nervous system.
- Deficiency symptoms – anaemia: fatigue, weakness, irritability, shortness of breath, spina bifida (if pregnant mother is deficient).
- Causes of deficiency – pregnancy, contraceptive pill, poor diet.

- Sources – wholegrains and green leafy vegetables.

Vitamin C

- Functions – necessary for healthy soft tissue and bones, wound healing and immune function.
- Deficiency symptoms – muscle aches and pains, stiffness after exercise, poor wound healing, bleeding gums, skin haemorrhages.
- Causes of deficiency – infections, stress, injury, old age (poor diet), smoking, drugs such as alcohol, barbiturates, antibiotics, corticosteroids and anti-inflammatories.
- Sources – fresh fruit and vegetables.

Calcium

- Functions – necessary for healthy bones, teeth, nerve and muscle function.
- Deficiency symptoms – muscle cramps, muscle and joint pain, growing pains, osteoporosis.
- Causes of deficiency – lack of exercise, old age, pregnancy, breast feeding, post menopause, children – especially during growth spurts.
- Sources – dairy products, canned fish, nuts, fruit, vegetables.

Calcium deficiency is a common cause of osteoporosis in the elderly (see chapter 2), particularly in post-menopausal women. It is a very common feature of old age as a result of a denatured diet and lack of exercise. The amount of calcium built up in the tissues before the age of 35 is important to prevent osteoporosis in later life. There is good evidence to show that supplementing calcium,

800–1,000mg per day, can delay the onset of osteoporosis in the elderly.

Iron

- Function – essential for transportation and storage of oxygen; necessary for function of enzymes and the immune system.
- Deficiency symptoms – anaemia; tiredness, lethargy, pale skin, breathlessness, giddiness, palpitations.
- Causes of deficiency – very common in women – heavy periods, pregnancy, breast feeding, poor diet.
- Sources – meat, egg yolks, green vegetables.

Iron deficiency is a very common symptom in women of child-bearing age and the major cause of anaemia. It can often occur in cases of internal bleeding from the gut. This can be caused by gastritis and stomach ulcers. A common cause of bleeding from the gut is the use of aspirin and anti-inflammatory drugs.

Magnesium and potassium

- Function – important for cell function, closely linked to calcium and sodium.
- Deficiency symptoms – weakness, loss of appetite, low blood pressure, cramps, irregular heartbeat, muscle weakness.
- Causes of deficiency – diarrhoea, laxatives, excessive salt intake, diuretics, poor kidney function, poor diet.
- Sources – nuts, wholegrains, green leafy vegetables and fruit.

Summary

Many nutritionists regard deficiency symptoms of these vitamins and minerals as being remarkably common. Good nutrition is vital to good health! A good intake of these nutritional factors will improve the recovery of someone suffering from musculoskeletal problems who may be mildly or borderline deficient. None of these vitamins or minerals is likely to have a toxic side effect when taken in doses commonly available in multivitamin and mineral preparations. If in doubt see your doctor or a nutritional therapist.

SMOKING

It has been well documented that smoking is a significant cause of cancer and heart disease. Smoking can be a factor in producing muscle fatigue and delaying muscle recovery following fatigue. It replaces a proportion of the oxygen in the blood with carbon monoxide, and as a result the fresh blood reaching the muscles is not of the quality it should be. Smoking has been linked to an increased incidence of pain and prolapsed discs in the lumbar spine. The mechanisms associated with this are considered to be:

- The strain of coughing.
- The association between smoking and diminished mineral content of bone.
- The reduction in quality of blood flow to the spine.

DIAPHRAGMATIC BREATHING

The diaphragm is a large dome-shaped muscle situated at the base of the rib cage. It separates the chest from the abdomen. The common slouched sitting posture compresses the chest and abdominal cavities, hindering the efficient function of the diaphragm as the main muscle of breathing. To compensate for this many people continually use the accessory muscles of breathing situated in the neck, shoulders and chest. This is a very inefficient form of breathing and can lead to fatigue and circulatory inefficiency. This is described in chapter 2 on pages 17–19.

Poor breathing technique is remarkably common, particularly when people are in pain or under stress. There is a simple exercise that can make you aware of good breathing technique and allow you to take advantage of more efficient functioning of your diaphragm.

- Stage 1 – Lie flat on the floor with a pillow underneath your head. Spend a minute or two allowing your body to relax, feeling the tension coming out of your neck and shoulders, your chest and pelvis, and your arms and legs.
- Stage 2 – Become aware of your breathing, make sure it is slow and relaxed. When you are first made aware of your breathing there is a tendency to breathe faster and deeper. Try to avoid this, maintaining a slow, relaxing breathing rhythm.
- Stage 3 – Place your hands on the upper part of your abdomen just below your ribs. As you breathe in watch your hands rise with your abdomen and fall as you breathe out. At this stage your abdomen should be the only part of your trunk that moves with breathing. Make sure the upper part of your rib cage is relaxed and still.
- Stage 4 – Place your hands on the lower part of the abdomen just below your navel and repeat stage 3.

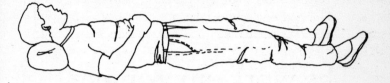

This is efficient diaphragmatic breathing, sometimes known as abdominal breathing. It's easy isn't it? In fact, although it sounds simple some people's bad habits of breathing are so ingrained that they find it very difficult to do at first. They have difficulty relaxing the accessory muscles of breathing and the chest continues to rise and fall with each breath. It shouldn't! Practise this for about five minutes every day for the first week or until you become accomplished at it. The next stage is to repeat stages 3 and 4 in the sitting position and ensure that you maintain your efficient breathing while seated. Once you have become aware of it, it becomes very easy to ensure that you are breathing properly in a variety of daily activities. Many people choose to continue this breathing exercise even after they have mastered it because it is a very pleasant relaxation technique – a good way to unwind after the completion of the day's work.

Efficient abdominal breathing is enhanced by a good upright sitting posture. The greater the angle between the trunk and the thighs (as in the forward-tilt seat) the less crowded the abdomen and the better the diaphragm is able to function.

11

The work environment

The ability to work efficiently depends on a comfortable harmonious environment that enables us to work without enduring distractions. There are a number of features that should be taken into account when planning your work environment and your working day.

FATIGUE

Most reductions in work efficiency are mediated by a state of fatigue. Fatigue can be isolated to a specific part of the body such as visual fatigue or muscular fatigue, or it can be a more generalised fatigue such as from overwork or lack of sleep. There are many factors that can determine at what point fatigue starts to develop. Some of these are unrelated to the work environment, such as health status, lack of sleep and domestic stress. In this section I am mainly concerned with the factors in the work environment that can be controlled and influenced in order to produce a good work environment, good work habits and to minimise the occurrence of fatigue.

Muscular fatigue

Muscular fatigue occurs after repeated use of a particular muscle group. It results in reduced power of muscle contraction, slower action and prolonged recovery period of the muscle. We can easily produce muscular fatigue by doing press ups or sit ups. It is more common in the sitting situation to produce muscular fatigue by poor posture or repetitive use. An example of poor posture is working with the head in a forward-bent position so that the muscles at the back of the neck become fatigued. An example of overuse fatigue is the extensor muscle strain at the wrist and forearm due to continual keyboard work without sufficient variation or breaks.

There is often a tendency to ignore fatigue or to be unaware of it due to the distractions that occur when working. It is important to become aware of when a muscle is likely to be fatigued and recognise the early stages to avoid the more serious problems that take place when fatigue becomes prolonged. The best way of avoiding muscular fatigue is by:

- Good ergonomics.
- Variation of tasks.
- Regular breaks (see page 249).

Generalised fatigue

The primary symptom of fatigue is the onset of weariness. This is not an unpleasant feeling if we are able to relax, but can be distressing if we have to push ourselves to meet deadlines. Weariness is a warning device like pain or hunger to discourage us from doing harm; to allow time for recovery. Fatigue is related to our state of arousal. If we have an interesting, stimulating job that we enjoy, we can delay the onset of fatigue. If we have a boring, monotonous, repetitive job, fatigue can set in rapidly.

Stress can often lead to a short-term arousal and an improvement of function, but when prolonged it produces a state of fatigue. Working under continual stress is known to be bad practice. It leads to fatigue, tiredness and an increased incidence of RSI, depression and chronic fatigue syndromes. These result in more absenteeism and a higher staff turnover.

People work best if they have some ability to control their work rate and take breaks or task variations when they feel it is appropriate. In the long term they become more productive and more content. Mental fatigue occurs when a task requires a high degree of concentration or vigilance. Examples of this are air traffic controllers and bus drivers. There are strict rules governing how many hours' work per day or the duration of work without a break for these occupations because it is well recognised that after a period of time there is a marked increase in the risk of error. This is a sign of fatigue.

FATIGUE CHECKLIST

Generalised fatigue can be avoided by:

- Interesting, varied tasks.
- Ability to work at own pace.
- Avoiding prolonged hours.
- Regular breaks.
- A low stress environment.

BREAKS

The concentration span varies with each individual, the task and the circumstances. It is generally regarded that the optimum attention span for most tasks is between 45 minutes and one hour. After this the concentration deteriorates, fatigue begins and work efficiency deteriorates. For vigilant tasks requiring a high degree of attention it can be down to 30 minutes, but for enjoyable and interesting tasks it can be over an hour.

The ideal time to take a break is just prior to the deterioration of concentration. A break taken here will produce a quick recovery and a renewed period of concentration. The break can be a change in task that allows the mental and physical faculties that have been utilised a period of rest. For example, after a period of office or computer work, using the photocopier or making a telephone call would be classed as a break. For jobs that involve continued attention without variation, such as a data operator, it is necessary that these breaks be scheduled at regular intervals. For jobs that allow varied tasks there can be a mixture of work variation and scheduled breaks. When left to our own devices, there is often a tendency to work beyond the optimum time for a break to reach a self-imposed cut off point, hence the importance of scheduled breaks and the awareness of efficient working practice.

Lengthy periods spent doing repetitive data processing are generally undesirable and an inefficient use of resources. A job that allows a variation of tasks is regarded as a more efficient working practice and leads to improved work satisfaction. It is becoming generally accepted that with tasks involving extensive VDU use, a break away from the screen of between five and 15 minutes in each hour is desirable. Active rest is more beneficial than passive rest. It is helpful to have a change in posture away from sitting and some active muscular movements to improve the circulation, stretch the muscles and enhance the process of recovery.

Many people seem to find working at a VDU screen has an addictive quality. They relentlessly work away ignoring breaks, ignoring fatigue and are seemingly unaware of passing time. This is very bad work practice and is likely to produce overuse problems. People who spend large portions of the day working at a keyboard should not be doing the same activity in the evenings and weekends as this does not allow sufficient recovery periods.

PAUSES

Pauses are short breaks that occur naturally during the working day. They can range from a few seconds to a few minutes. Spontaneous pauses are pauses for rest that workers take on their own initiative, such as chatting to a colleague or using the bathroom.

Disguised pauses are opportunities the worker takes to do an easier task in place of their normal more demanding job. It might be cleaning the VDU screen or going for a walk to get some stationery. These pauses are common and have an important function. They help people regulate their work rate and control the degree of fatigue. There is a general tendency to make more pauses in the last two hours of the working day when the level of fatigue is greater. It is important to recognise that these pauses are a legitimate part of good work practice. Where there are more prescribed breaks, it is often found that employees are less fatigued and take fewer pauses as a result. For this reason, having regular prescribed breaks can actually lead to an improvement in work efficiency and a greater work output.

As well as being aware of the necessity of breaks and pauses, it is a good idea to take maximum advantage of them by performing some exercise or postural variation. When you are waiting for your computer to process information, lean back in your chair and have a good stretch. While you are talking on the phone it is easy to do some wrist or neck stretching exercises. I encourage my patients who drive a lot to do some upper body exercises while their vehicles are in traffic jams or at traffic lights.

THE WORKING DAY

The typical working day is seven and a half or eight hours long, the working week being 35 to 40 hours. More varied working practices are becoming popular, with flexitime, job sharing and part-time work proving to be a good use of resources and popular with many employees.

Overtime is still commonplace. Increasing the working day beyond eight hours can often produce a drop in total work output as the fatigue that develops leads to a slower overall work rate. In addition, it can lead to a higher absentee rate due to sickness and accidents. Generally speaking, working extended hours is not productive.

Working through lunch or tea breaks in order to shorten the working day is not something that is desirable. It would be expected to lead to early onset of fatigue and reduced efficiency and quality of work.

The appropriate amount of time spent each day working at a VDU screen is a contentious issue and most commentators choose not to commit themselves to a figure. It can certainly be a highly variable recommendation based on the nature of the work, the quality of the work station and the personal characteristics of the worker, such as age, experience, work rate, personality, etc. However, as the world we live in becomes increasingly computerised and many conventional jobs are being changed to become computer bound, often with little thought given to the ability of the worker to cope, I believe it is important to establish some guidelines. Five hours per day is the maximum time that a worker should be expected to spend at a VDU screen. This should be broken up into segments throughout the day as opposed to being continuous blocks and should be interspersed with a 10 minute break every hour.

A WORK SCHEDULE

This is a suggested working schedule when working at a computerised work station, based on an eight-hour day with one hour for lunch.

Hours	Time working	Breaks
1	50 minutes' computer work	10 minute
2	50 minutes' computer work	10 minute
3	1 hour non-computer work	
4	1 hour computer work	
5	lunch	
6	50 minutes' computer work	10 minute
7	1 hour non-computer work	
8	50 minutes' computer work	10 minute
9	1 hour non-computer work	

This allows for five one-hour segments of computer work, each with a break incorporated or immediately following. There is only one block of two hours' continuous computer work which has a 10 minute break after 50 minutes and another after 110 minutes.

With employees who are new to a job or who are returning after an absence due to sick leave or holiday, it is desirable that they be gradually phased in to the normal working schedule and intensity.

Each break should include some physical activity. If appropriate, it is a good idea to include some of the key exercises or the three-minute upper body stretch in the breaks (see page 230). When planning your working schedule, it is worthwhile being aware of the known factors that can increase the possibility of fatigue. These are:

- Increasing age.
- Increased experience.
- Previous accident or overuse injury.
- Quality of work station.
- Stress levels.
- Work rate – faster work rate produces earlier fatigue.

EYE STRAIN

Eye strain or visual fatigue results from doing visually demanding tasks for long periods. It is often brought on by unsatisfactory viewing conditions. The symptoms of eye strain are usually brought on by overuse of the muscles around the eye. Working at a VDU screen is known to be particularly visually demanding. There are a number of studies that describe 60 to 80 per cent of VDU users complaining of visual difficulties. The symptoms of eye strain include:

- Irritation – redness, dryness, itching, watery eyes.
- Visual disturbance – difficulty in focusing, blurriness.

- Headaches – usually frontal or behind the eyes, sometimes with nausea and dizziness.

The visual demands of working at a computer often show up eye defects that were previously unrecognised, and unless corrected, the eyes become rapidly fatigued. Contact lens wearers can have problems with eyes drying out and becoming irritated.

Eye testing

If a job requires habitual use of a VDU it is wise to have an eye assessment prior to commencing work. This will ensure that any weaknesses can be accommodated and the appropriate measures taken to prevent eye strain. A further test should be taken after a few months to ensure that no eye problems are developing. Further tests should be taken at regular intervals or whenever eye strain becomes apparent. The Health and Safety Regulations provide for the cost of eye testing to be met by the employer.

Glasses

Bifocals are normally designed for reading and writing at distances of 300–500mm. Most VDU users prefer distances greater than this and it may cause difficulty for the users of bifocals. The solution is to have glasses made for the focal distance required. The Health and Safety Regulations provide for the employer to cover the cost of corrective appliances (glasses) required for display screen work. The provision of glasses for any other viewing distances such as reading or distance vision is the responsibility of the individual. The employer's liability is limited to the cost of a basic appliance.

Users of bifocals often hold an awkward head and neck position to ensure vision through a particular part of the lens. This can produce neck strain and headaches. The solution is to have corrective glasses suitable for the visual demands of the task. While it is acknowledged that using a VDU can cause eye strain, there is no evidence that it causes permanent damage. The eye strain can respond quickly to adequate rest and so it is important to ensure that regular breaks are taken away from the screen to reduce the effects of visual fatigue.

LIGHTING

Research has shown that in many workplaces productivity can rise and the error rate fall by improving the quality of lighting. Lighting levels are dependent on the visual acuity required for the task. General guidelines are:

- Moderately precise – packing, carpentry, engineering: 200–300 lux.
- Fine work – reading, writing, book-keeping: 500–700 lux.
- Precision work – technical drawing, sewing, delicate electronics: 1,000–2,000 lux.

For general office work a range of 500–700 lux is considered appropriate. For VDU work the desirable range is 300–500 lux. Overbright lighting (over 1,000 lux) can lead to visual strain caused by reflections, glare, contrast between light and shadow, etc. The lux level can easily be measured using a hand-held device available from lighting and electrical specialists.

General guidelines for lighting

- Walls should be light coloured to allow an even distribution of light.
- Sharp contrasts between dark flooring or furniture and reflective table tops should be avoided.
- It is better to use more lamps of low power than a few very bright ones.
- No light sources should be visible in the visual field when working.
- Light sources should never flicker.
- Lighting sources (windows and lights) should be placed at right angles to the work station rather than directly in front or behind.
- Glare from windows can be reduced by using blinds or tinted film.

Glare, reflections and sharp colour contrasts can be visually disturbing and lead to visual fatigue. Good placement of lights and windows is important. A light source behind the operator can cause a reflected glare from a VDU screen. A light source in front can produce direct glare. Ceiling or wall lights can be shielded to reduce the amount of direct lighting. Uplighting, which produces an indirect light source, can be helpful.

NOISE

Noise levels are best kept to a minimum. Main sources of noise in the office are fans and printers. Printers tend to be the most annoying noise and this can be overcome by housing them separately or converting to an inkjet or laser printer, both of which are noiseless. The noise level should be below 65 decibels, and if a high degree of concentration is required, below 55 decibels.

TEMPERATURE

Comfort levels of temperature are subject to considerable personal variation. These can be influenced by:

- Clothing.
- Posture.
- Fat levels.
- Individual metabolic rate.
- Personal preference.

Variations in temperature can lead to levels of discomfort which can inhibit good work practice and productivity. It is important to keep a relatively constant, comfortable environment. Sedentary work does not produce a great deal of body heat, so the working environment preferred is one that is warmer than an environment for manual work. The recommended air temperature is 20 to 21°C in summer and 20 to 24°C in winter. No single surface should be in marked contrast to the air temperature. Draughts can be an irritating factor to a sedentary worker. They can create local muscle spasms that can inhibit the efficiency of work and can lead to muscle fatigue. The head, neck and feet are particularly sensitive to draughts. Cold draughts are more irritating than warm draughts. Adequate heat control and ventilation is a better way of controlling excessive heat than fans.

HUMIDITY

The range of humidity that is comfortable is 30 to 60 per cent. If the humidity drops to below 30 per cent and the air becomes too dry there is an increase in respiratory tract problems such as sinusitis, bronchial irritation and infections of the nose and throat. Pot plants and humidifiers can help to increase the humidity.

RADIATION

The emission or transfer of radiant energy as particles, electromagnetic waves, sound, etc. *Collins English Dictionary*

Most electrical equipment emits low dosages of radiation when in use. Whether prolonged exposure to low dosages of radiation can be harmful to health is not yet fully understood and is the subject of considerable research and scientific debate.

In the early 1980s there were concerns that full-time work at a VDU caused an increased risk of abortion and birth defects in pregnant women. These concerns were fuelled by reported clusters of miscarriages and birth defects occurring in certain regions and workplaces. Larger studies have not consistently confirmed these findings.

A recent study in Finland (Lindbohm et al., 1992) found that women who worked with VDUs with high magnetic field levels (over 9 mG) in the Extremely Low Frequency (ELF) range, had over three times as many miscarriages as those exposed to less than 4 mG. Women exposed to 4 to 9 mG (ELF) had nearly twice as many miscarriages. This study of 191 women who had previously miscarried was one of the few studies to measure the level of radiation being emitted by computer terminals rather than the length of time sitting at a terminal.

Recent research published in 1992 (Ryan et al.) found

that women using cathode ray tube monitors (this includes most computers) have five times the number of brain tumours compared to women not using them. There have also been concerns that prolonged exposure to electromagnetic radiation may be a factor in leukaemia and breast cancer.

It would seem, therefore, that the health care concerns relating to the computerisation and electrification of the modern office are justified. These concerns are echoed in the Health and Safety (Display Screen Equipment) Regulations 1992, which state:

> All radiation with the exception of the visible part of the electromagnetic spectrum shall be reduced to negligible levels from the point of view of the protection of operators' or users' health and safety.

Kim Uildriks, a computer health care consultant gives the following advice to avoid unnecessary exposure to electromagnetic radiation:

- Position monitors carefully. Most radiation comes out of the rear and sides of a unit. Desks arranged back to back or at right angles can expose operators to someone else's radiation.
- Keep at least 1 metre from the front of the screen and at least 2 metres from the back or sides of a monitor.
- Keep at least 1 metre from other electrical equipment.
- Turn off the computer (and other electrical equipment) when not in use.

- Use anti-radiation shielding.
- If you are pregnant or planning a pregnancy and have concerns about the effects of VDU radiation, take the above precautions or ask to be transferred to non-VDU work. Alternatively use a low radiation monitor or a portable computer which has lower radiation levels.

Older monitors tend to have higher levels of radiation than more recent models. If purchasing a new monitor look for one that meets the Swedish recommended standards for radiation emissions.

12

Your action plan

Review your work station

- Fill in the work station assessment.
- Take a close look at your sitting position. Are there easy adjustments that you can make to your chair, desk, screen, etc?
- Regularly review your posture for the task that you are doing.
- Do you need a new chair or copy holder?

Seek help

- Discuss the situation with your employer or supervisor.
- Talk to your doctor.
- Have appropriate treatment if required.
- Get specialist ergonomic advice if necessary.

Plan your working day

- Ensure you get adequate job variation, with frequent postural change.
- Take regular scheduled breaks.
- Develop low stress work habits.

Stretching exercises

- Spend 10 minutes twice a day doing exercises that you have identified as being beneficial for you.
- Develop a two- to three-minute exercise programme incorporating the key exercises that you can do regularly throughout the day e.g. the three-minute upper body stretch on page 230.

Get fit

- Find a form of regular exercise that suits you.
- Start cautiously once a week.
- Aim to get some form of exercise each day with good aerobic exercise at least three times per week.

Relax

- Make sure you are able to relax muscle groups that are affected by overuse.
- Use relaxation exercises and techniques to help release tension and reduce stress levels.
- Ensure that you have a good diaphragmatic breathing pattern.

Control your weight – be healthy

- Follow a sensible wholefood diet with emphasis on fruit, vegetables and fish.
- Be careful of snacking.
- Restrict use of stimulants and alcohol.

ACTION PLAN FOR EMPLOYERS

This information is based on the requirements of the Health and Safety (Display Screen Equipment) Regulations 1992.

Work station analysis

- Make an assessment of each work station for each person using that work station.
- If you ask each employee to fill out the work station assessment in the appendix, this should identify any problems or areas that could be improved.
- Seek specialist help if necessary.
- Keep good written records.

Work station changes

- In consultation with your employees make the appropriate changes that you have identified.
- Consult individually with each employee as their requirements will not be identical.
- Keep written records of any improvements made.

Plan the work schedule

- Identify any jobs that require intensive VDU operation.

- Devise a work plan that gives job variation and regular breaks.
- Develop a low stress work environment.
- Make special provisions for staff returning after a period away from work.

Eye tests

- Find a good optician and come to an agreement regarding the provision of eyesight tests, eye examinations and supply of glasses.
- Ensure that each member of staff has an initial examination on commencing employment, on further request or when any problems arise.

Early warning system

- Develop a reporting system so that employees are able to report early signs of fatigue or discomfort. This enables overuse problems to be dealt with in their infancy.
- Ensure appropriate changes are made to the work environment and medical assistance is available when required.

Health and safety education

- Develop a programme of health and safety training.
- Provide an information package for each employee outlining the employer's obligations and the measures taken to comply with the Health and Safety Regulations.

CHOOSING YOUR OFFICE FURNITURE

The chair

It is important to find a good-quality chair that suits you in your work environment. It is worthwhile shopping around to see which you prefer and test driving a few to determine what your requirements are.

Don't set your heart on finding a bargain. The quality of the chair can be an important determinant of your ability to work effectively. When comparing the cost of a chair to your annual earning capacity, it is not an expensive item.

If you will be using the chair for more than two hours per day you should have an office type chair. It should swivel and it should be height adjustable. This ensures ease of mobility, variations of posture and ease of getting up and down.

The chair base

The chair should have a stable five-star base. It should not have a tendency to tip if you lean backwards or to one side. It should be on castors to improve ease of movement. On an uncarpeted floor, glides or castors with built-in friction are preferable.

The seat

The seat should be contoured with a rounded front edge. This will avoid any pressure points or restriction of circulation to the legs. It should be covered with 3 to 5cm of high-density foam. Soft foam will not provide adequate support. It should be upholstered with cloth, which helps to prevent a build up of heat and moisture and provides a degree of friction. Leather and particularly vinyl are not as suitable.

A forward-tilt seat provides definite advantages for the posture of the lumbar spine and pelvis and it is worthwhile giving serious thought as to whether you would benefit from this. The forward tilt can either be fixed, variable or adjustable. The forward tilt should be at least 5°, but can be up to 10°. A range of −5° to +10° forward tilt provides a maximum range of comfortable sitting postures.

Seat height

The seat height should be adjusted to provide the ideal relationship with the work surface. It should be at the appropriate height for a comfortable posture of the upper spine, shoulders and arms.

The next priority is to find a good leg position. If the feet cannot be comfortably placed on the floor, a foot stool should be used. If the knees are higher than the hips, as may be the case with very tall people, both the chair and the work surface should be raised. If both the work surface and the seat are height adjustable, then the chair can be adjusted for good leg position and the work surface adjusted for good upper body posture.

Back rest

The back rest should help maintain a lumbar curve in the normal working posture. It is worthwhile trying a chair while working to ensure that it is able to do this. The back rest should be adjustable for height and pivot. There should be at least 10cm between the base of the back rest and the seat, and the back rest should be adjustable up and down by at least 10cm. A small, well-positioned and contoured back rest will provide perfectly good back support for the upright working posture. For a reclined working posture, which is often favoured by VDU workers, a high well-shaped back rest is preferable. It should have good lumbar support and extend to the mid-spine, between the shoulderblades. It should not impede movement of the arms or shoulders. It should recline in the range from vertical to 30° backwards. A back rest should be able to be fixed in a degree of tilt, rather than being spring loaded.

Arm rests

Arm rests can be a useful addition to a chair providing they do not interfere with the positioning of the chair or the movement of the arms and shoulders. They can give valuable support with certain tasks and getting on and off the chair. They should not extend more than 250mm in front of the back rest and should be adjustable or removable in case they become inconvenient.

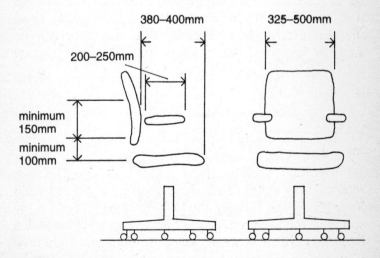

Fig. 12.1 Recommended seat dimensions.

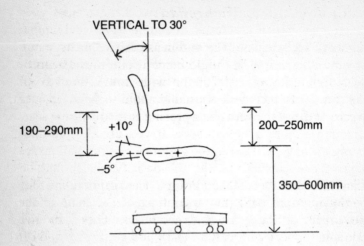

Fig. 12.2 Recommended seat adjustability.

Foot rest

A foot rest should be used if your feet are not able to sit comfortably on the floor when the chair is adjusted for optimum posture. It should be large enough to allow a variety of foot postures. It should be stable and in a horizontal position or slanted backwards up to 10°. You can experiment with books and planks of wood to determine a comfortable height and position and then buy a permanent foot rest or have one made. Too often people are inclined to muddle along with an old cardboard box or similar. See the photograph on page 95 for a good example of a foot rest.

Work surfaces

The work surface should be as thin as practicable to ensure maximum leg room. It should be non-reflective. The knee room should be at least 700mm wide and 550mm deep. The standard office desk is usually about 720mm high. If you are taller than average, or prefer a forward-tilting seat, you may require a higher desk. If you are shorter than average you will either require a foot rest or you will prefer a lower desk height. Ideally the desk height should be adjustable between 640 to 780mm. The main criterion of the desk height is to allow a comfortable neck, shoulder and arm working posture. This is determined by the following:

When sitting with the shoulders relaxed and the elbows at 90°, the work surface should be about 5cm above the bottom of the elbow. When typing or using a keyboard the platform should be at the height of the elbow, with the depth of the keyboard bringing the actual work surface up to the recommended height.

When using a keyboard the working height is critical to good shoulder, elbow and wrist posture.

For reading and writing tasks, an angled work surface produces significantly reduced strain to the neck, shoulders and upper spine. For writing the appropriate degree of tilt is 10 to 20°. For reading this can be increased to 45 to 60°. A good compromise for both functions is 15 to 25°. The sloping work surface can be built into the worktop and can be made to adjust to the required angle. Alternatively, an additional platform can be placed on the worktop when required.

WORK ASSESSMENT QUESTIONNAIRE

Use this questionnaire to help you determine the quality of
your work space and whether any alterations are required.
This will be valuable information for someone assisting
you in improving your work space, such as your employer
or occupational health nurse.

WORK ASSESSMENT QUESTIONNAIRE

1. What is your occupation?

2. How many hours of the working day do you
   spend sitting?

3. How many hours per day do you spend at a VDU?

4. Do you take regular breaks? How often and for
   how long?

5. Is your work environment comfortable for the
   following?
   - Lighting.
   - Temperature.
   - Humidity.
   - Air conditioning.

6. Do you have any difficulties with glare or reflection?

7. How would you describe the stress levels at
   work?
   - Low.
   - Medium.
   - High.

8. How would you describe the content of your work? Boring, repetitive, monotonous, varied, interesting, stimulating, challenging.

9. Is your chair height adjustable?

10. Does your chair have a forward-tilt mechanism? If not, would you prefer a chair with a forward-tilt option?

11. Does the back rest adjust for height and tilt?

12. Are you able to use the back rest in your normal working posture?

13. When working at your comfortable work height are your feet able to sit comfortably on the ground? If not, do you have a foot rest that allows you to place both feet flat, with sufficient space to vary your foot position?

14. Do you have sufficient leg room?

15. Is your desk at a comfortable working height? If not, is it possible to make alterations to your desk height?

16. Is there sufficient space for you to arrange your work comfortably?

17. Do you use a backward-tilted work surface for reading and writing tasks? If not, would you benefit from using one?

18. Are the following joints able to find a comfortable working position?
    • Shoulders.
    • Elbows.
    • Wrists.
    • Neck/head.

19. Is the keyboard separate from the screen?

20. Is the keyboard at a comfortable working height?

21. Is the keyboard height adjustable?

22. Is there sufficient space in front of the keyboard for wrist support?

23. Is the screen clear and easy to read?

24. Is the screen adjustable for height, tilt and depth?

25. Is a copy holder provided at your work station? If there is, do you use it regularly?

HEALTH ASSESSMENT QUESTIONNAIRE

This is to help you assess whether you are suffering from any work-related health problems. This information will be helpful to your doctor or anyone who is helping with these symptoms.

HEALTH ASSESSMENT QUESTIONNAIRE

1. Do you suffer from any of the following? Tick as appropriate.

                              Never   Sometimes   Often

Low-back pain
Mid-back pain
Neck or shoulder pain
Upper arm pain
Elbow pain
Wrist or forearm pain
Finger or hand pain
Hip or pelvic pain
Leg or ankle pain
Pins or needles, numbness
Muscle weakness
Eye strain
Headaches/migraines
Stress
Depression
Frustration

Mark on the anatomical chart (overleaf) your areas of pain.

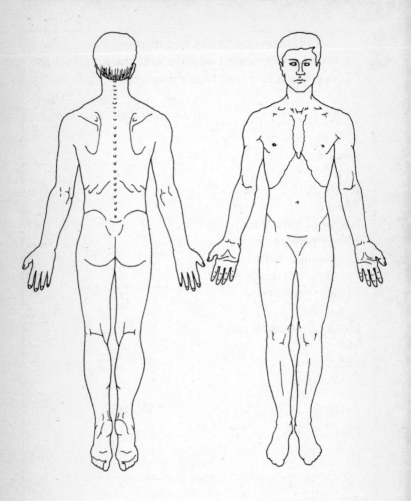

2. List your areas of pain and discomfort, approximately how long you have had them and what
   you think may have been the cause.

                    Location   Duration   Cause

   1.

   2.

   3.

   4.

   5.

   6.

   7.

   8.

   9.

   10.

3. Have you had to take any time off work as a result
   of these complaints?

4. Describe any activities that make your symptoms
   worse.

5. Describe any activities that relieve your symptoms.

6. Do these problems have any effect on your private life e.g. housework, sport, leisure activities? Describe.

7. Do these problems affect your sleep?

8. How would you describe the amount of stress involved with your work?
   • High.
   • Moderate.
   • Low.

9. How would you describe the amount of stress in your private life?
   • High.
   • Moderate.
   • Low.

10. Do you enjoy your work?

11. If you have work-related fatigue or overuse problems, have you discussed them with your employer?

13

Some case histories

CASE 1

Ms M. began to develop pain, stiffness and swelling in her right arm in mid-1987. Her job as a legal secretary involved mainly writing and typing. Her natural diligence and desire to complete her legal executive qualifications often meant long hours with a high work rate.

She sought medical assistance and was given anti-inflammatory medication and a course of physiotherapy. The condition gradually worsened despite treatment. It spread to her left arm and began to affect her home life. The pain turned to agony, sleeping became very difficult and routine household tasks became an ordeal. She had to give up her interests such as waterskiing, ten-pin bowling and knitting.

In December 1988, her GP advised six weeks off work and when she returned it was on the understanding that she would not have to type. It was unsuccessful. In March 1989, Ms M. left work permanently. She was in constant pain, she had to curtail her leisure activities severely and abandon her promising career as a legal executive.

After nearly 12 months off work, her employer, who had remained supportive, re-employed her as a receptionist/ telephonist on a reduced income. She continued to have considerable difficulty but was able to modify her work-place and plan her work so that she was able to continue with the assistance of therapy. She was unable to do much writing and completely unable to type. She was only able to work due to the understanding of her employers. Her confidence and self-esteem were naturally affected by her limited work prospects and restricted private life.

Ms M. is one of the unfortunate cases that occurred in the mid-1980s when there was less understanding of the causes of RSI and the importance of early recognition and modification of the workplace. Despite frequent medical attention, a strong work ethic and a concerned employer, her condition progressed to the point where work was no longer possible and her enjoyment of life was dramatically diminished by pain and disability.

Nearly four years later Ms M.'s life is still overshadowed by the looming presence of RSI constantly reminding her of its existence and the importance of managing her life to avoid the progression of pain. I can do no better than let her describe her current situation:

1993
Over the years I've had gradual improvement. I'm still aware of a certain amount of pain and dis-comfort every day of my life, but for the first time this year I'm doing legal secretarial work again. I work two hours per day. Initially I had quite a lot of pain and discomfort, but as the weeks passed by my hands settled down again. With anything that's new I find this happens. I found a similar

thing happened when I had a newborn baby to take care of. I'm not doing a great deal of typing and never will again. What typing I'm doing is in short bursts. If I do have to do anything that is straight copy typing and consists of several pages, I take this home and break it up into 15 minute sessions.

RSI is something that can't be seen physically, which is why there are a lot of non-believers, but it is something that rules every day of your life. Even to write these few lines, I feel pain and discomfort. I still have swollen areas, but I have come a long way from the days of having to have someone else to cut my meat and my mum coming over to do my housework, and even using one arm at a time to wash my hair.

I've always enjoyed working hard no matter what, and I've always been determined to put my life back together as best as I can, which I believe I have done, and you get used to a certain amount of pain and discomfort in your day.

It is easy to recognise in hindsight the problems that lead to Ms M.'s condition: the lack of a height-adjustable chair, a high work surface, an excessively high keyboard, her tendency to overwork and a delayed initiation of appropriate medical management. It must be placed in the context of the information that was available at the time and the widespread ignorance of the true causes of RSI.

We must learn from cases such as hers to take immediate and appropriate preventive measures when the early symptoms become apparent so as to prevent more victims of this modern disease.

CASE 2

Soon after Ms A. came to me for treatment, it became apparent that although her RSI symptoms were improving she would not be able to return to her job as a receptionist at a large medical centre.

She first developed RSI symptoms in 1990 when working as a medical dictaphone typist. It started in her left thumb, spreading to her left wrist and forearm and then to her right arm. She sought treatment and found relief of pain with anti-inflammatories and physiotherapy, but as soon as she returned to keyboarding the same gripping pain came rushing back. She tried using wrist splints and she tried acupuncture. She consulted a rheumatologist and then a consulting physician who gave her three cortisone injections into her carpal tunnel. None of these gave her any significant relief.

Ms A. eventually had to give up work. She continued to have acupuncture and other therapy and began to make a good recovery. After six months off work she was re-employed at the medical centre as a telephonist and was able to cope with a limited amount of keyboard work. After a few months she left her home town and travelled for two years, doing a variety of reception and secretarial jobs with no further difficulties.

She returned after her adventures and started work as a medical receptionist in the same practice she had worked in previously. After a month of full-time work her symptoms returned in full force, affecting both arms and also her neck and shoulders. She struggled on trying to find a way of coping with the pain, but within a few months she was forced to give up work again. With osteopathic treatment and a home treatment and exercise programme her pain and disability have diminished substantially, though she remains unable to use a keyboard.

With the permission of her employer I undertook an assessment of her work station. It showed what are probably the three most common faults in VDU work.

- Work surface and keyboard were too high.
- There was inadequate wrist support.
- The screen was too low. It had annoying reflections.

Ms A. had a supportive employer and was given a wide range of quality medical care. But there seemed to be a reluctance to seek and implement the specialised advice needed to improve the ergonomics of her work place and as such the major cause of her problems remains unchanged.

She has made good progress with treatment and her pain is almost disappeared. She has been off work for four months.

CASE 3

RSI is not confined to the workplace. The following case is that of a student who experienced a similar reluctance by the institution she attended to recognise the seriousness of her problems and an inability to deal effectively with the cause.

Ms H. started to feel the aching, gripping pain in her left forearm six weeks after she began studying architecture. Initially it was just when she used her ruler for drawing. It gradually extended to causing pain in her everyday life. Then it spread to her right arm, developing into a continuous burning pain whenever she used her hands.

Ms H. consulted her GP. He suggested some physiotherapy treatment and anti-inflammatory medication. This gave some relief and she was able to complete her assessments, but it was only temporary. The pain continued to spread and began to affect her neck and shoulders. After six months she began to have pain at night and difficulty sleeping. She had to withdraw from her studies.

Ms H. is a 23-year-old Danish girl. She consulted me after 18 months of continuous pain. She was by then working as an au-pair and studying languages, but still suffered considerable discomfort on a daily basis. She is tall, with long limbs and a long neck. She has generally hypermobile ('loose') joints with weak muscle tone. This is a hereditary characteristic which makes her more prone to overuse injuries as she does not have a great deal of strength to cope with continued postural stress. She showed a gradual improvement with treatment and I showed her how to treat herself on a daily basis using ice and massage. I explained the principles of good posture and how to reduce the stress of prolonged sitting. I outlined the importance of regular exercise to improve her muscle tone.

I treated Ms H. once a week for eight weeks and she showed steady improvement. We were hopeful that on her return to Denmark she would be able to resume her studies. She was keen to study English literature.

I was disappointed to learn that the school of architecture was quite unhelpful with her problem to a point of denying that it was related to her studies. It is a shame that there is such a poor understanding of postural considerations in an institution that is training the next generation of architects.

In each of the three cases above the unfortunate sufferer has had to give up work or study. I have tried to identify some of the reasons why the problems developed and how the severity could have been avoided. The next two cases show how with effective management, the person has been able to continue employment. Effective management usually involves:

- Early recognition of the problem.
- An understanding employer who is prepared to make the appropriate alterations to the work station and to the work routines.
- Appropriate medical advice and therapy.

CASE 4

Ms N. first noticed pain in her wrists following a marked increase in her word processing workload as part of her role as a receptionist/secretary in a bank. Typing became difficult and the keys seemed to be heavier than they used to be. The pain spread to her forearms and started to impact upon her home life. Her employers were sympathetic and understanding and she was taken off all typing and transferred to other office duties. She was sent for medical assessment to her GP who advised rest and therapy.

After six weeks Ms N. was able to return to a limited amount of word processing and with a sympathetic employer she was able to manage her workload carefully.

Her reception desk was in a busy office traffic area and not well designed as a computer work station, with the keyboard being significantly higher than recommended. The strain on her arms and shoulders was reduced by using an Ergorest forearm support (see the illustration on page 91) which she found very helpful.

Five months after the initial injury she had a recurrence of RSI symptoms in a more acute form so that she was unable to hold a pen. It was at this point she consulted me about osteopathic treatment. I explained to her the ergonomic and postural principles and the importance of regular breaks. We developed a home treatment and exercise programme for her. She was able to continue work through this episode, but had to be very careful in her work management.

> The improvements (the forearm supports), ensuring that I do my exercises regardless of how busy I am, and the osteopathic treatment have helped my arms tremendously. I do get a few twinges and have bad days if the workload is too much. With understanding employers it does make life a bit easier.

CASE 5

Ms J. arrived for treatment with a 'screaming' headache. It began one month previously when she lifted a piece of timber and had been present ever since despite various methods of treatment. She had become tense and distressed.

Ms J. responded well to her first treatment and by the following day the headache had cleared. Over the next 10 days it gradually returned complete with neck and shoulder spasms. It became clear that this was part of a work-related overuse strain, not just a single injury.

She had worked in a legal firm as a typist for the last six years. During this time they had changed from typewriting to word processing with a VDU screen. She worked at the screen for eight hours every day. They had recently reduced their office staff and she took particular pride in her ability to manage the increased workload and continuously maintain a very high work rate.

After consultation with her specialist we decided to reduce her hours, so she was working half her normal time while we continued with therapy. Initially this improved her symptoms. But after a few weeks she began to get quite distressed about being unable to work her normal hours. She felt frustrated and under-utilised and she started to develop some anxiety symptoms about being on part-time work. She seemed to be suffering some type of work withdrawal symptoms.

Ms J. had one further week with intensive treatment at a residential facility and then returned to full-time work. She promised me that she would not work more than five hours at a VDU screen each day; take a 10 minute break each hour; and use a copy holder more often. She would try to work at a more relaxed pace.

Her employer had been co-operative and had allowed her to reduce her workload and plan her day to schedule more regular breaks. When I last spoke to her she was working well, without any significant problems.

The next two cases illustrate how people suffering from low-back pain can benefit from using a forward-tilt chair.

CASE 6

Ms L. has a history of recurrent spinal problems following previous injuries. She has had a career as a book-keeper and has successfully made the transition from a manual workplace to a computerised workplace.

After recently being made redundant she decided to become self-employed, assisting small businesses to keep good financial records. She found the stress of being self-employed and the continual postural demands of computer operation intensified her spinal problems. She found the stress–tension–pain cycle aggravated her problems, making it difficult to work efficiently. She became depressed and frustrated with her work.

I reviewed her work habits and the ergonomics of her work station with her and I suggested she replace her dining chair she used for computer work with an office chair with a forward tilt of 10°. This enabled her to work more efficiently and with much reduced muscle tension and back pain. She recently wrote to me:

> Thank you for the opportunity to purchase this most amazing chair on which I sit. It makes such a tremendous difference, one could hardly credit it.

CASE 7

Mr B. is a successful businessman, the managing director of his own company. After a week of being at his desk he enjoys a physically active weekend. It was after one of these that he arrived at my clinic on Monday morning, unable to stand straight and in considerable pain. We were able to treat him, but the injured disc in his spine remained too sensitive for any weight bearing, so he was sent home for rest.

After two days he was able to stand and walk for limited periods, but found sitting very painful. He was unable to sit in his office chair, but found he was much more comfortable sitting in a kneeler chair. We lent him a kneeler chair and he was able to resume work to a limited capacity. He borrowed the kneeler chair for the next three weeks while his back remained sensitive, after which he was able to return to his conventional office chair. The kneeler chair allowed him to return to his managerial duties much sooner than he would otherwise have been able to. He was able to be more productive and reduce his pain and disability by using the kneeler chair during his recovery period.

Mr B. made a full recovery and was able to resume his normal seating. Many similar cases, after a serious back injury, choose to use or have ready access to a forward-tilt chair or a kneeler chair.

CASE 8

Ms B. began to develop neck stiffness soon after starting secondary school. It seemed to be aggravated by school work. The neck pain spread to affect her shoulders and upper back and she began to get frequent headaches. She noticed the headaches became worse during the typing class.

For the first 18 months she used pain killers when they were needed and her parents frequently massaged her neck. Over the period of exams, her headaches and neck stiffness became worse and it became difficult for her to concentrate. When she realised she was having headaches every day, she decided with her parents that it was time to seek professional help.

I explained to Ms B. how poor posture when studying can lead to neck tension and headaches. I explained the principles of good posture and the benefits of working at a sloping desk. Following treatment she felt much better and I demonstrated some exercises to prevent her neck stiffening up again. Her parents made her a desk for home study with a 30° slope.

I needed several treatments from the osteopath and have felt much better since. He showed me techniques to relieve the tension myself, including using a sloping desk at home. I get some tension returning during exams when we have a lot of pressure and have to sit for long periods.

Sitting has become a feature of our modern life, and many of us do not associate the health problems that we develop with the sitting that we do. This book establishes clear links between health problems and sitting, and provides the information to avoid or minimise these problems. This knowledge gives us the ability to influence these areas of our lives, and to take appropriate preventive measures to reduce the risk of these health problems. Listen to your body and try to recognise problems before they become serious, and act accordingly. Take personal responsibility for your health!

The world can only be grasped by action, not by contemplation ... The hand is the cutting edge of the mind.

Jacob Bronowski

Appendix

A summary of the Health and Safety (Display Screen Equipment) Regulations 1992 (Crown copyright. Reproduced with the permission of the Controller of Her Majesty's Stationery Office). The conditions described in the regulations came into force on 1 January 1993.

Regulation 1 – Deals with definitions described under the Regulations. It describes which employers and what types of equipment are covered.

Regulation 2 – Requires employers to analyse and assess the health and safety risks of each work station. It requires them to reduce the risks identified to the lowest extent reasonably practicable.

The assessment should be reviewed when there is a change in the user or the user's capability, a change in the work station or a change in the job requirement.

Regulation 3 – Details the timing of the regulations.

- All work stations put into service on or after 1 January 1993 must meet the requirements as described.
- All work stations put into service on or before 31

December 1992 must meet the requirements not later than 31 December 1996.

Regulation 4 – Requires that daily work on display screen equipment be periodically interrupted by breaks or changes of activity. It gives guidance on the nature and timing of these breaks.

Regulation 5 – Requires that an eye and eye sight test be provided by the employer for the employee on commencement of work at a VDU screen and at regular intervals. When an employee experiences visual difficulties which may reasonably be considered to be caused by display screen equipment, he or she should be provided with an appropriate eye and eye sight test on request. Any corrective appliances (spectacles) required specifically for display screen work should be provided by the employer.

Regulation 6 – Requires that all employees be provided with adequate health and safety training in the use of work stations upon which they may be required to work.

Regulation 7 – All employees must be provided with adequate information about all aspects of safety relating to their work stations and measures taken by the employer in accordance with these regulations.

THE SCHEDULE

This is reproduced in full and sets out the minimum health and safety requirements for work with display screen equipment. The extent to which employers must ensure that work stations meet the requirements is laid down in this Schedule.

1. An employer shall ensure that a work station meets the requirements laid down in this Schedule to the extent that:
   (a) Those requirements relate to a component which is present in the work station concerned;
   (b) those requirements have effect with a view to securing the health, safety and welfare of persons at work; and
   (c) the inherent characteristics of a given task make compliance with those requirements appropriate as respects the work station concerned.

Equipment

2. (a) *General comment* – The use as such of the equipment must not be a source of risk for operators or users.
   (b) *Display screen* – The characters on the screen shall be well defined and clearly formed, of adequate size and with adequate spacing between the characters and lines.

   The image on the screen should be stable, with no flickering or other forms of instability.

   The brightness and the contrast between the characters and the background shall be easily adjustable by the operator or user, and also be easily adjustable to ambient conditions.

   The screen must swivel and tilt easily and freely to suit the needs of the operator or user.

   It shall be possible to use a separate base for the screen or an adjustable table.

   The screen shall be free of reflective glare and reflections liable to cause discomfort to the operator or user.

(c) *Keyboard* – The keyboard shall be tiltable and separate from the screen so as to allow the operator or user to find a comfortable working position avoiding fatigue in the arms or hands.

The space in front of the keyboard shall be sufficient to provide support for the hands and arms of the operator or user.

The keyboard shall have a matt surface to avoid reflective glare.

The arrangement of the keyboard and the characteristics of the keys shall be such as to facilitate the use of the keyboard.

The symbols on the keys shall be adequately contrasted and legible from the designated working position.

(d) *Work desk or work surface* – The work desk or work surface shall have a sufficiently large, low-reflectant surface and allow a flexible arrangement of the screen, keyboard, documents and related equipment.

The document holder shall be stable and adjustable and shall be positioned so as to minimise the need for uncomfortable head and eye movements.

There shall be adequate space for operators or users to find a comfortable position.

(e) *Work chair* – The work chair shall be stable and allow the operator or user easy freedom of movement and a comfortable position.

The seat shall be adjustable in height.

The seat back shall be adjustable in both height and tilt.

A foot rest shall be made available to any operator or user who wishes one.

Environment

3. (a) *Space requirements* – The work station shall be dimensioned and designed so as to provide sufficient space for the operator or user to change position and vary movements.

   (b) *Lighting* – Any room lighting or task lighting provided shall ensure satisfactory lighting conditions and an appropriate contrast between the screen and the background environment, taking into account the type of work and the vision requirements of the operator or user.

   Possible disturbing glare and reflections on the screen or other equipment shall be prevented by co-ordinating workplace and work station layout with the positioning and technical characteristics of the artificial light sources.

   (c) *Reflections and glare* – Work stations shall be so designed that sources of light, such as windows and other openings, transparent or translucid walls, and brightly coloured fixtures or walls cause no direct glare and no distracting reflections on the screen.

   Windows shall be fitted with a suitable system of adjustable covering to attenuate the daylight that falls on the work station.

   (d) *Noise* – Noise emitted by equipment belonging to any work station shall be taken into account when a work station is being equipped, with a view in particular to ensuring that attention is not distracted and speech is not disturbed.

   (e) *Heat* – Equipment belonging to any work station shall not produce excess heat which could cause discomfort to operators or users.

(f) Radiation – All radiation with the exception of the visible part of the electromagnetic spectrum shall be reduced to negligible levels from the point of view of the protection of operators' or users' health and safety.

(g) *Humidity* – An adequate level of humidity shall be established and maintained.

Interface between computer and operator/user

4. In designing, selecting, commissioning and modifying software, and in designing tasks using display screen equipment, the employer shall take into account the following principles:

(a) software must be suitable for the task;

(b) software must be easy to use and, where appropriate, adaptable to the level of knowledge or experience of the operator or user; no quantitative or qualitative checking facility may be used without the knowledge of the operators or users;

(c) systems must provide feedback to operators or users on the performance of those systems;

(d) systems must display information in a format and at a pace which are adapted to operators or users;

(e) the principles of software ergonomics must be applied, in particular to human data processing.

For a full copy of these regulations and further guidance on the regulations, contact:

HMSO Publications Centre
PO Box 276
London SW8 5DT
Telephone orders: 071 873 9090
Fax orders: 071 873 8200

or HMSO Bookshops.

Useful addresses

The General Council and Register of Osteopaths
56 London Street
Reading
Berkshire
RG1 4SQ
0734 576585

The British Medical Association
BMA House
Tavistock Square
London
WC1H 9JP
071 387 4499

General Medical Council
44 Hallam Street
London
W1N 6AE
071 580 7642

The Royal College of General Practitioners
14 Princes Gate
Hyde Park
London
SW7 1PU
071 581 3232

British Orthopaedic Association
Royal College of Surgeons
35 Lincoln's Inn Fields
London
WC2A 3PN
071 405 6507

Institute of Orthopaedics
Royal National Orthopaedic Hospital Trust
45–51 Bolsover Street
London
W1P 8AQ
071 387 5070

The National Back Pain Association
The Old Office Block
Elm Tree Road
Teddington
Middlesex
TW11 8ST
081 977 5474

The British Osteopathic Association
8–10 Boston Place
London
NW1 6QH
071 262 5250

British Chiropractic Association
29 Whitley Street
Reading
Berks
RG2 0EG
0734 757557

UNITED STATES
American Osteopathic Association
300 Fifth Street North East
Washington DC 20007
United States
(202) 544 5060

American Physical Therapy Association
1111 North Fairfax Street
Alexandria
Virginia 22314
United States
(703) 684 2782

CANADA
Canadian Osteopathic Association
575 Waterloo Street
London
Ontario N6B 2R2
(519) 439 5521

AUSTRALIA
Occupational Health and Safety Council
Cnr Spencer St and Flinders St
Melbourne 3000
Telephone 628 8111

Worksafe
Level 4,
400 Kent St
Sydney 2000
Telephone 370 3503

Australian Osteopathic Association
1/267 Castlereagh Street
Sydney,
NSW 2000
Telephone 02 264 9171

Ergonomic Society of Australia
Canberra Business Centre
Bradfield Street
Downer
ACT 2602
Telephone 242 1951

NEW ZEALAND
Occupational Safety and Health
PO Box 3705
Wellington
Telephone 471 2937

Accident Compensation Corporation
Private Bag,
Wellington
Telephone 473 8775

New Zealand Register of Osteopaths
PO Box 11 853
Wellington

New Zealand Ergonomics Society
PO Box 802
Palmerston North

Bibliography

BOOKS

Anderson B., *Stretching*, Pelham Books, 1980.

Baldry P.E., *Acupuncture, Trigger Points and Musculoskeletal Pain*, Churchill Livingston, 1989.

Bogduk N., Twomey L.T., *Clinical Anatomy of The Lumbar Spine*, Churchill Livingston, 1987.

Bullock M.I. (editor), *Ergonomics: The Physiotherapist in the Workplace*, Churchill Livingston, 1990.

Caillet R., *Hand Pain and Impairment*, F.A. Davis Company, 1975.

Caillet R., *Shoulder Pain*, F.A. Davis Company, 1966.

Caillet R., *Soft Tissue Pain and Disability*, F.A. Davis Company, 1977.

Corrigan B., Maitland G.D., *Practical Orthopaedic Medicine*, Butterworths, 1983.

Department of Labour, New Zealand, *Code of Practice For Visual Display Units*, 2nd edition, 1988.

Fisk J.W. , *Fitness For All Ages*, Charles C. Thomas, 1984.

Fisk J.W., *Your Painful Neck and Back*, Century Hutchinson, 1987.

Fisk J.W., *Medical Treatment of Neck and Back Pain*, Charles C. Thomas, 1987.

Grandjean E., *Fitting the Task to the Man*, 4th edition, Taylor and Francis, 1988.

Hartley A., *Practical Joint Assessment*, Mosby-Year Book, Inc., 1990.

Health and Safety Executive, *Seating at Work*, London: HMSO, 1991.

Health and Safety Executive, *Display Screen Equipment Work, Health and Safety (Display Screen Equipment) Regulations 1992*, HMSO, 1992.

Kapandji I.A., *The Physiology of the Joints*, volume 3, Churchill Livingston, 1974.

Kirkaldy-Willis W.H., *Managing Low Back Pain*, 2nd edition, Churchill Livingston, 1988.

Kisner C., Colby L.A., *Therapeutic Exercise*, 2nd edition, F.A. Davis Company, 1990.

Kulund D.N., *The Injured Athlete*, 2nd edition, J.B. Lippincott Company, 1988.

Lucie-Smith E., *Furniture: a Concise History*, Thames and Hudson, 1979.

Magee D.J., *Orthopaedic Physical Assessment*, W.B. Saunders Company, 1987.

Mandal A.C., *The Seated Man: Homo Sedens*, Dafnia Publications, 1985.

National Occupational Health Information Service, New Zealand, *Seating for Office Workers*, Department of Health, 1989.

Norkin C.C., Levangie P.K., *Joint Structure and Function*, F.A. Davis Company, 1992.

O'Brien W., *An Employer's Guide to the New VDU Legislation*, Sven Christiansen PLC, 1992.

Occupational Safety and Health, New Zealand, *Occupational Overuse Syndrome. Treatment and Rehabilitation: A Practitioner's Guide 1992*; *Occupational Overuse Syndrome. Guidelines For Prevention and Management 1991*, Department of Labour.

Pheasant S., *Ergonomics, Work and Health*, MacMillan, 1991.

Travell J.G., Simons D.G., *Myofascial Pain and Dysfunction: The Trigger Point Manual*, volume 1, Williams and Wilkins, 1983.

Travell J.G., Simons D.G., *Myofascial Pain and Dysfunction: The Trigger Point Manual*, volume 2, Williams and Wilkins, 1992.

Zacharkow D., *Posture: Sitting, Standing, Chair Design and Exercise*, Charles C. Thomas, 1988.

JOURNALS

Adams M.A., Hutton W.C., 'The Effect of Fatigue on the Lumbar Intervertebral Disc', *Journal of Bone and Joint Surgery*, 65B: 199–203, 1983.

Adams M.A., Hutton W.C., 'The Effect of Posture on the Fluid Content of Lumbar Intervertebral Discs', *Spine*, 8: 6, 665–671, 1983.

Adams M.A., Hutton W.C., 'Gradual Disc Prolapse', *Spine*, 10: 524–531, 1985.

Andersson G.B.J., 'Loads on The Spine During Sitting', *Ergonomics of Working Posture*, eds Corlett, Wilson, Manenica. Proceedings of First International Occupational Ergonomics Symposium, 309–318, 1985.

Bendix A., Jensen C.V., Bendix T., 'Posture, Acceptability and Energy Consumption on a Tiltable and a Knee Support Chair', *Clinical Biomechanics*, 3: 66–73, 1988.

Bendix T., 'Seated Trunk Posture At Various Seat Inclinations, Seat Heights and Table Heights', *Human Factors*, 26:6, 695–703, 1984.

Bendix T., 'Chair and Table Adjustments for Seated Work', *Ergonomics of Working Posture*, eds Corlett, Wilson, Manenica. Proceedings of First International Occupational Ergonomics Symposium, 355–362, 1985.

Bendix T., Biering-Sorensen F., 'Posture of the Trunk When Sitting on Forward Inclined Seats', *Scandinavian Journal of Rehabilitative Medicine*, 15: 197–203, 1983.

Bendix T., Bloch I., 'How Should a Seated Workplace With a Tiltable Chair be Adjusted?', *Applied Ergonomics*, 17:2, 127–135, 1986.

Bendix T., Hagberg M., 'Trunk Posture and Load on the Trapezius Muscle Whilst Sitting at Sloping Desks', *Ergonomics*, 27:8, 873–882, 1984.

Bendix T., Winkel J., Jessen F., 'Comparison of Office Chairs with Fixed Forwards or Backwards Inclining, or Tiltable Seats', *European Journal of Applied Physiology*, 54:4, 378–385, 1985.

Bennett R.M., 'Myofascial Pain Syndromes and the Fibromyalgia Syndrome: a Comparative Analysis', *Journal of Manual Medicine*, 6:1, 34–45, 1991.

Corlett E.N., Eklund J.A.E., 'How Does a Backrest Work?', *Applied Ergonomics*, 15:2, 111–114, 1984.

Corlett E.N., McAtamney L. 'Ergonomics in the Workplace', *Physiotherapy*, 74:9, 475–478, 1988.

Drury C.G., Francher M., 'Evaluation of a Forward Sloping Chair', *Applied Ergonomics*, 16:1, 41–47, 1985.

Eklund J.A.E., Corlett E.N., 'Experimental and Biomechanical Analysis of Seating', in *Ergonomics of Working Posture*, eds Corlett, Wilson, Manenica, Proceedings of First International Occupational Ergonomics Symposium, 317–330, 1985.

Eklund J.A.E., Corlett E.N., 'Evaluation of Spinal Loads and Chair Design in Seated Work Tasks', *Clinical Biomechanics*, 2:1, 27–33, 1987.

Fisk J.W., Baigent M.L., Hill P.D., 'Scheuermann's Disease: a Clinical and Radiological Survey of 17 and 18 year olds', *American Journal of Physical Medicine*, 63, 18–30, 1984.

Grieco A., 'Sitting Posture: An Old Problem and a New One', *Ergonomics*, 29:3, 345–362, 1986.

Grandjean E., Hunting W., 'Ergonomics of Posture – Review of Various Problems of Standing and Sitting Posture', *Applied Ergonomics*, 8:3, 135–140, 1977.

Grandjean E., Hunting W., Nishiyama A., 'Preferred VDT Workstation Settings, Body Posture and Physical Impairments', *Applied Ergonomics*, 15:2, 99–104, 1984.

Jelenski G., 'An Investigation Into the Occurrence and Prevention of Cumulative Trauma Disorders of the Upper Limbs and Neck in Medical Laboratory Scientific Officers', thesis for Diploma in Osteopathy, British College Of Naturopathy and Osteopathy, 1991.

Jensen C.V., Bendix T., 'Spontaneous Movements with Various Seated-Workplace Adjustments', *Clinical Biomechanics*, 7:2, 87–90, 1992.

Lander C., Korbon G.A., DeGood D.E., Rowlingson J.C., 'The Balans Chair and its Semi-kneeling Position: An Ergonomic Comparison with the Conventional Sitting Position', *Spine*, 12:3, 269–272, 1987.

Lee S., 'Repetitive Strain Injury – The Issue and the Enigma', *Journal of Osteopathic Education*, 3:2, 76–78, 1993.

Life M.A., Pheasant S.T., 'An Integrated Approach to the Study of Posture in Keyboard Operation', *Applied Ergonomics*, 15:2, 83–90, 1984.

Lindbohm M.L. et al., 'Magnetic Fields of Video Display Terminals and Spontaneous Abortion', *American Journal of Epidemiology* 136:9, 1041–1051, 1992.

Mandal A.C., 'Investigation of the Lumbar Flexion of Office Workers', in *Ergonomics of Working Posture*, eds Corlett, Wilson, Manenica, Proceedings of First International Occupational Ergonomics Symposium, 345–354, 1985.

McIlwraith B., 'An Analysis of the Driving Position in the Modern Motor Car', *British Osteopathic Journal*, 11: 27–33, 1993.

Official Journal of the European Communities, 'Council Directive on the Minimum Safety and Health Requirements for Work with Display Screen Equipment', L 156: 14–18, 29 May 1990.

Ryan P., Lee M.W., North B.J., McMichael, A.J., 'Risk Factors for Tumours of the Brain and Meninges', *International Journal of Cancer*, 51: 20–27, 1992.

Simons D.G., 'Myofascial Pain Syndrome and Fibromyalgia' (editorial), Muscle Pain Syndromes, *Journal of Manual Medicine*. 6:1, 1–23, 1991.

Stoddard A., Osborn J.F., 'Scheuermann's Disease or Osteochondrosis: its Frequency and Relationship with Spondylosis', *Journal of Bone and Joint Surgery*, 61B: 56–58, 1978.

Uildriks K., 'Computer Health', *Options*, March 70–71, 1992.

Uildriks K., 'Computer Health Hazards', *Options*, October 56–58, 1993.

Wilson A., 'The Incidence of Spinal Complaints in College Students – a Preliminary Report', *Journal of the New Zealand Register of Osteopaths* 6: 16–17, 1993.

Winkel J., Jorgensen K., 'Evaluation of Foot Swelling and Lower Limb Temperatures in Relation to Leg Activity During Long-Term Seated Office Work', *Ergonomics*, 29:2, 313–328, 1986.

Zaidi L., 'An Osteopathic and Ergonomic Analysis of the Visual Display Unit', thesis for Diploma in Osteopathy, British College of Naturopathy and Osteopathy, 1991.

Index